'97

Nurse–Midwifery Handbook

A Practical Guide to Prenatal and Postpartum Care

Nurse–Midwifery Handbook

A Practical Guide to Prenatal and Postpartum Care

Linda Wheeler, CNM, EdD

Oregon Health Sciences University
Portland, Oregon

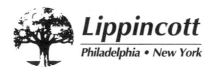

Lippincott

Philadelphia • New York

Acquisitions Editor: *Jennifer E. Brogan*
Editorial Assistant: *Susan V. Barta*
Project Editor: *Barbara Ryalls*
Production Manager: *Helen Ewan*
Production Coordinator: *Nannette Winski*
Design Coordinator: *Kathy Kelley-Luedtke*
Indexer: *Victoria Boyle*

9 8 7 6 5 4 3 2 1

Library of Congress Cataloging in Publications Data

Wheeler, Linda A.
Nurse–midwifery handbook: a practical guide to prenatal and postpartum care/by Linda Wheeler.
    p. cm.
Includes bibliographical references and index.
ISBN 0–397–55360–9 (alk. paper)
    1. Midwifery. 2. Prenatal care. 3. Postnatal care. I. Title.
RG950.W48 1997
618.2—dc21   96–49608
                                                                              CIP

Care has been taken to confirm the accuracy of the information presented and to describe generally accepted practices. However, the authors, editors, and publisher are not responsible for errors or omissions or for any consequences from application of the information in this book and make no warranty, express or implied, with respect to the contents of the publication.

The authors, editors and publisher have exerted every effort to ensure that drug selection and dosage set forth in this text are in accordance with current recommendations and practice at the time of publication. However, in view of ongoing research, changes in government regulations, and the constant flow of information relating to drug therapy and drug reactions, the reader is urged to check the package insert for each drug for any change in indications and dosage and for added warnings and precautions. This is particularly important when the recommended agent is a new or infrequently employed drug.

Some drugs and medical devices presented in this publication have Food and Drug Administration (FDA) clearance for limited use in restricted research settings. It is the responsibility of the health care provider to ascertain the FDA status of each drug or device planned for use in their clinical practice.

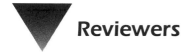 **Reviewers**

Marie Brown, CNM, PNP, PHD
Oregon Health Sciences University
Portland, Oregon

Virginia L. Capan, CNM, MA
University of New Mexico Health Sciences Center
Albuquerque, New Mexico

Linda D. Glenn, CNM, PMHNP, MN, MPH
Orgeon Health Sciences University
Portland, Orcgon

Christine Heritage, MS
Cottage Grove Women's Health Care
Cottage Grove, Oregon

Carol Howe, CNM, DNSc
Oregon Health Sciences University
Portland, Oregon

Richard Lowensohn, MD
Oregon Health Sciences University
Portland, Oregon

Kathleen Murray, CNM, MS
Franciscan Midwives at St. Joseph's
Tacoma, Washington

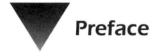

Preface

Welcome to the circle of midwifery. At the center is the mother and her baby. A step away is the mother's family and others with whom she is intimately connected. Farther away is the community to which she belongs and into which she brings her baby. Looking in and attending all are the health professionals who protect and care for this woman.

Nurse–Midwifery Handbook: A Practical Guide to Prenatal and Postpartum Care is a result of my attempts to help novice practitioners enter the midwifery circle. It suggests a framework for combining art and science as students begin work in the clinical area. Hints are provided on how to gather data, interpret it, and, in conjunction with the client and her family, follow a course of action that is safe, nurturing, respectful, and caring. This book is neither a textbook nor a cookbook. Rather, it is a guide that gives suggestions on how to ask questions and provides a framework for being thorough. *The suggestions are meant to be tried on—to see what fits and what does not fit.* Not everything will be useful. Not every approach will feel right. Methods of diagnosis and treatment vary from one community to another. As you read, ask yourself, "Is that true?" "Will that work?" "Is this something I should try in my own practice?"

Many of us feel passionately about various issues—the "right way" to do a pelvic examination, the role of nutrition in pregnancy, the best way to feed a baby. Unfortunately, good evidence for many common practices is often absent or conflicting. It may be helpful to remember that much of what we do is culturally determined ritual and may not be based in fact, but also may not consider the needs of an individual woman. These cultural paradigms, whether or not they are based on research, are powerful determinants of practice.

As clinicians, we must read professional journals on a regular basis and make every attempt to base our practice on valid evidence. Critical reading of research articles involves some knowledge of the research process so that appropriate conclusions about the value and validity of the research can be made. A helpful guide for evaluating obstetrical research is *A Guide to Effective Care in Pregnancy and Childbirth* (Enkin, M., Keirse, M.J.N.C., Renfrew, M., & Neilson, J., 1995, (2nd ed.), New York: Oxford University Press, $23.00). This book was written to disseminate to clinicians the conclusions of a systematic review of published and relevant unpublished controlled trials in perinatal medicine and is an important addition to midwifery practice.

Clinicians must also observe, listen, and question. We should reflect often on our practice and the many influences upon it. The ability to understand these influences is an important step toward maturity as a clinician.

We have a common goal—the birth of a healthy baby to a healthy mother in a manner that keeps the power of choice within the center of the circle. The wise practitioner knows that we differ in our approaches, our beliefs, our fears, and our confidence. There is no *one* way to be a midwife. Regardless of professional affiliation, each should aspire to embrace the tenets of midwifery, for the word means "with woman". Enter the circle with awe and respect, with hope and with kindness. Bring your presence, your experience, your wisdom. Readers are invited to send me their own thoughts about good prenatal and postpartum care so that the many valuable but different approaches can be shared with others.

I am grateful to Christine Heritage, CNM, MS, Carol Howe, CNM, DNSc, and Richard Lowensohn, MD, for reading and critiquing various parts of this book. Special thanks to Virginia Capan, CNM, MA; Linda Glenn, CNM, PMHNP, MPH, MN, and Kathleen Murray, CNM, MS who read the entire manuscript and generously shared their words and their wisdom. Special, special thanks to Marie Brown, CNM, PNP, PhD, who read at least three versions of the manuscript.

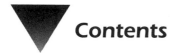

Contents

▼ PART 3   The Prenatal Revisit   91

▼ PART 4   The Postpartum Period   149

Preconception Counseling

While most pregnancies in the United States are unplanned, there are many individuals who carefully consider the many factors that might affect the outcome of pregnancy before attempting to conceive. Some of these people will schedule a visit with a health care provider for preconception counseling to discuss the genetic, medical, obstetrical, behavioral, environmental, and psychosocial factors that could pose a problem for either mother or baby should pregnancy occur.

Preconception counseling also provides an opportunity to discuss laboratory testing that may be indicated to assist in an assessment of risk, as well as an opportunity to discuss readiness for parenting. Should a pregnancy be decided upon and achieved, preconception counseling allows for discussion of the kind of birth experience that will best meet the needs and desires of the family. It should also include a review of the factors that optimize pregnancy outcome.

▼ Successful Interviewing

The chances for a productive initial interview are increased when good communication skills are used. This means attending to those aspects of the physical environment that are in your control and asking questions in a way that invites the client to share parts of her life with you. The way you ask questions, the words you use, your tone of voice, expressions of interest—all will influence how much she will tell you. Other ways to facilitate interviewing include allowing the client to finish her thoughts in her own words without interruption and waiting until she is finished before saying, "Tell me a little more about . . ." Encourage the expression of feelings.

Maximize privacy. Eliminate interruptions, including disturbances by other health care personnel and intrusions of a pager or beeper. Be aware of personal mannerisms that may be distracting to others. For example, frequent use of "okay," "uh," and "basically" as well as head nodding can be annoying to clients. The obstacles you will encounter include time constraints imposed by the workplace, your own fears and resistance (feeling intrusive, embarrassed, helpless, wanting to fix things), and reservations on the part of the client. Respect her decisions about what she will share.

Also respect personal cultural proscriptions. Be aware of the potential for violating "boundaries" with physical contact. A hug, for example, may be frightening to a woman who has been sexually abused. In fact, women with a history of sexual abuse may not wish any unnecessary physical contact from the clinician.

▼ The History

Family History

The family history is obtained to identify couples who may be at risk for having a child with a birth defect. "A birth defect is an abnormality of structure, function, or body metabolism which often results in a physical or mental handicap, shortens life, or is fatal. It may be inherited or may result from environmental interference within the womb or from outside" (March of Dimes). Race and ethnic background and a family medical history can help determine whether or not genetic counseling is indicated. The family history can also provide information about psychiatric illness in either parent, as well as parental or sibling use of alcohol and illicit drugs, factors that increase the chances that the client (or her partner) experienced childhood neglect or abuse. Sensitive recognition of these issues is often appreciated by individuals thinking about parenting.

Racial and Ethnic Background

Ask about the racial and ethnic background of the potential parents so that carrier testing for conditions that are more prevalent in certain racial and ethnic groups can be offered. Thalassemia, the most common genetic disease, occurs worldwide but most frequently in people from West and Central Africa, the Mediterranean basin (Italy, Sicily, Greece, North Africa), the Middle East, South Asia, Southeast Asia, Southern China, and the Pacific Islands. Testing for the thalassemia begins with a complete blood count.

Family Medical and Obstetrical History

The family medical history at a preconception visit is intended to identify significant inherited disorders in first-degree (parents, siblings, children) and second-degree (grandparents, grandchildren, aunts and uncles, nieces and nephews) relatives. Three or more miscarriages in a first-degree relative may indicate a chromosome translocation. A baby may be stillborn because of an unrecognized genetic disorder. A neonatal death may be due to an inherited metabolic disorder. A baby who died early in life may have died from sudden infant death syndrome (SIDS) but also may have had a genetic disorder, particularly in the case of atypical SIDS (death before 1 month of age or after 12 months) or multiple deaths attributed to SIDS. Mental retardation in a family member may represent a heritable form of mental retardation, Fragile X syndrome being the most common. Mental retardation is most significant when two or more family members are affected and/or the retardation is associated with dysmorphic features.

Important information can be obtained by asking questions about the father of the baby and his family history. In addition to racial and ethnic background, ask if his family has a history of mental retardation, a birth defect, a genetic disorder, or a chromosome abnormality. Ask, as well, if he has been involved in any relationship in which three or more miscarriages have occurred. Order a karyotype of any man who was the father of three babies that were miscarried. Appendix A contains sample genetic history questions.

Diethylstilbestrol

Ask a potential mother born before 1974 if she knows whether or not her mother used any medicine to keep from miscarrying when the client was in utero. Diethylstilbestrol (DES), a drug used until the early 1970s to prevent miscarriage and other complications of pregnancy, is associated with increased vaginal and cervical cancer, as well as variations and structural abnormalities in the cervix and vagina of daughters who were in utero when their mothers were treated with DES. DES daughters also have increased rates of infertility, abortion, ectopic pregnancy, and preterm labor.

Preeclampsia

Preeclampsia, a disease unique to pregnant women, has a small but significant incidence of recurrence when a mother or sister has had severe preeclampsia. Ask about problems with high blood pressure during pregnancy in the client's mother or sister(s).

Mental Illness

Ask also about a family history of mental illness, as some psychiatric disorders—schizophrenia, depression, and bipolar disease, for example—have hereditary components. Additionally, living with or in close association with someone with a mental disease can be difficult. Life may be unpredictable and chaotic. A sick parent may have been unavailable for basic physical and emotional needs. When mental illness exists in the family, it may be helpful for the clinician to ask about fears the client may have about personal mental illness or its development in her child. It is also appropriate to inquire about the effect that a family member's mental illness may have had on the client's life. Since emotional and psychiatric problems often are not officially diagnosed, also ask the client if depression or unstable and unexpected behavior was present in any family member.

Alcohol and Drugs

Parental abuse of alcohol or use of illicit and recreational drugs often leads to neglect or abuse of children. Therefore, include questions about past and present use of alcohol or drugs in family members. Not only does violence occur frequently in families with substance abuse problems, but physical and emotional nurturing may have been lacking. Life may have been chaotic as parents struggled to support their habit, maintain a home, and keep or find a job. Multiple foster care placements involving repeated separation and loss may have occurred. Try asking "How much alcohol did your parents use when you were growing up? How often did they drink? What about drugs? How often did they smoke marijuana? How about other drugs? How often did they use them? Did your brothers and sisters use?"

When it is evident that substance abuse has occurred, ask "How old were you when this was happening?" and "What was it like for you growing up in that environment?" It is rare that individuals who grew up in families where substance abuse was common escape without some emotional sequelae. Parents-to-be often appreciate acknowledgment of the difficulties these situations may have caused.

Personal Medical History

Maternal Age

Pregnancy, labor, and birth are safest in most respects when a baby is born to a mother between the ages of 20 and 34. Both younger (aged 13 to 17) and older (aged 18 or 19) teenage mothers have an increased chance of delivering premature and growth-retarded babies. The problems encountered by older pregnant women (aged 35 and older) are usually a result of chromosomal abnormalities (Table 1-1) or the medical complications from chronic illness that are more likely to occur as women get older. Medical problems contribute to the older gravida's greater risk for spontaneous abortions, premature separation of the placenta, intrauterine growth restriction, macrosomia (abnormally large baby), and stillbirth. The incidence of preterm delivery is increased because labor is induced more often for maternal medical problems and small-for-date babies. Fortunately, treatment is available for many women with chronic disorders, and the absolute number of stillborn babies is low.

TABLE 1-1. Risk of Chromosomal Abnormality (at birth)
at Various Maternal Ages*

Maternal Age	Risk for Down Syndrome	Total Risk for Chromosomal Abnormalities†
20	1:1667	1:526
21	1:1667	1:526
22	1:1429	1:500
23	1:1429	1:500
24	1:1250	1:476
25	1:1250	1:476
26	1:1176	1:476
27	1:1111	1:455
28	1:1053	1:435
29	1:1000	1:417
30	1:952	1:385
31	1:909	1:385
32	1:769	1:322
33	1:602	1:286
34	1:485	1:238
35	1:378	1:192
36	1:289	1:156
37	1:224	1:127
38	1:173	1:102
39	1:136	1:83
40	1:106	1:66
41	1:82	1:53
42	1:63	1:42
43	1:49	1:33
44	1:38	1:26
45	1:30	1:21
46	1:23	1:16
47	1:18	1:13
48	1:14	1:10
49	1:11	1:8

* Because sample size for some intervals is relatively small, 95% confidence limits are sometimes relatively large. Nonetheless, these figures are suitable for genetic counseling.

† 47 XXX excluded for ages 20–32 (data not available) (Source: American College of Obstetricians and Gynecologists. *Antenatal diagnosis of genetic disorders.* Technical Bulletin No. 108. Washington, DC: ACOG ©1991. Reprinted with permission.)

Women who will be 35 years of age or older at the birth of their baby should be offered genetic counseling and prenatal testing with chorionic villus sampling or amniocentesis. When older women without chronic disease carry a chromosomally normal baby, clinicians can be optimistic about the outcome of pregnancy (Cunningham & Leveno, 1995).

Organic Disease

Certain medical conditions have the potential for affecting the mother or baby, or both. A prospective mother needs to know that her own disease may worsen or may increase the chances that a baby would be sick or die. Below are some medical conditions in this category.

Epilepsy

Most epileptic women find that pregnancy has no effect on their disease. Some even experience an improvement. Those who find that their disease worsens are likely to be women with severe disease (Wilhelm, Morris, & Hotham, 1990). Compared with nonepileptics, women with epilepsy have a two- to threefold increased risk of giving birth to a child with malformations (Cunningham et al, 1993) and a 2% to 3% risk of having a child with a seizure disorder. They are also at increased risk for preeclampsia and preterm labor.

Women with epilepsy are often taking anticonvulsant medicine when they become pregnant. Phenytoin (Dilantin) is commonly used. When taken during pregnancy, this drug is associated with the fetal hydantoin syndrome—intrauterine growth retardation, microcephaly, facial abnormalities, developmental delays, and mental retardation. The exact contribution of phenytoin to fetal abnormalities is unknown, as it is difficult to distinguish between the disease and the medicine, or a combination of each. Hemorrhagic disease of the newborn may occur in the babies of some pregnant women who take phenytoin. Parenteral vitamin K given to the baby immediately after birth prevents these coagulation defects.

Insulin-Dependent Diabetes Mellitus (IDDM)

Many years ago few women with diabetes were able to conceive. Those who did become pregnant experienced high rates of fetal loss. Stillbirth was common. The advent of insulin made motherhood possible for diabetic women, but the road to a healthy baby without maternal morbidity can be difficult, especially for women with poorly managed or difficult-to-control diabetes.

Women with IDDM may develop severe hypertension, preeclampsia, ketoacidosis, and even blindness and renal failure. Excessive amniotic fluid may develop. The fetus is at increased risk for congenital abnormalities and may be unusually large or small (intrauterine growth restriction). If the baby is macrosomic, vaginal delivery can be traumatic to both mother and baby. Difficulty delivering the baby's shoulders can lacerate maternal tissue and damage the baby's arm and clavicle. Postpartum hemorrhage is more likely to occur. Women with IDDM should be followed by an obstetrician or perinatologist when possible.

Hypertension

Women with chronic hypertension are at increased risk of having preeclampsia, preterm delivery, and a growth-retarded baby. Premature separation of the placenta (abruptio placenta), with its potential for both maternal and fetal morbidity and mortality, is more likely to occur. Physician management of this condition is preferred, as medicine to control blood pressure is likely to be needed or adjusted. Special tests to assess fetal growth and well-being are indicated.

Cancer

Although spontaneous abortion is increased in cancer survivors, the risk of cancer to their offspring is not increased unless a parent carries a cancer susceptibility gene. A woman who has had cancer is likely to ask about her risk for a recurrence of the cancer as well as the child's risk for cancer. These women should be referred to a genetic counselor who can help an individual woman evaluate her risk. Congenital malformation rates after radiation and chemotherapy do not seem to be increased (Schneider, 1994).

Lupus Erythematosus

The effect of systemic lupus erythematosus (SLE), a multisystem disease, on pregnant women is variable. Some women experience no new problems. This is particularly true if the disease has been in remission at least 6 months before conception. Other women experience an exacerbation of symptoms with hospitalization required. Spontaneous abortion, intrauterine growth restriction, preterm delivery, congenital cardiac defects, and perinatal death may occur. A recent study of pregnant women with lupus showed a 50% prematurity rate, with 39% of these women experiencing premature rupture of the membranes as well (Johnson, 1995).

Tuberculosis

In developed countries tuberculosis is not more serious in pregnant women than in nonpregnant women. However, drug resistance has become a serious problem in the United States, and the increase in human immunodeficiency virus (HIV) infection, as well as immigration from countries where tuberculosis is endemic, has significantly increased the rate of tuberculosis. While drugs used for treatment do pose risks to the fetus and neonate, treatment is essential, the risk of tuberculosis outweighing the risk of drug toxicity (Davidson, 1995).

Screening for tuberculosis is appropriate for a woman who is:

Symptomatic
HIV positive
A close contact of a person with pulmonary tuberculosis
An alcoholic or IV drug user
From a country with a high prevalence rate
A resident of a correctional institution or a long-term care facility
A health care worker
Poor and medically underserved.

Prior vaccination with bacillus Calmetter-Guerin (BCG) vaccine should not preclude a tuberculin skin test for anyone who received this vaccine in infancy or childhood because sensitivity decreases 10% per year without repeated doses.

Thyroid Disease

Both hypo- and hyperthyroid disease can pose problems for mother and baby. Women with hyperthyroidism are at increased risk for preeclampsia and heart failure. Their babies may have neonatal thyrotoxicosis and die in utero.

Hypothyroidism is rarely a problem in pregnancy as long as a woman continues to take thyroid medication, usually levothyroxine. Without appropriate medicine, however, the newborn may develop hypothyroidism.

Heart Disease

Cardiac disease contributes substantially to maternal death. Pregnancy is contraindicated in certain cardiac diseases, and a decision about whether or not to attempt pregnancy when cardiac disease is present is best made in conjunction with a perinatologist and a cardiac specialist.

Hematological Disorders

Some anemias have health implications for both mother and baby. For example, some of the thalassemias are associated with preterm labor, intrauterine growth restriction, and increased fetal loss. Babies with thalassemia may face severe anemia, failure to thrive, and premature death. Sickle cell trait increases the risk of urinary tract infection in pregnant women, but women with other sickle cell hemoglobinopathies may have chronic debility and a shortened life span.

Women with hematologic problems, as well as women with the potential of passing these medical problems on to their offspring, need consultation with a perinatologist before making a final decision about whether or not to attempt pregnancy. Often the father of the baby should be tested to identify the nature and extent of the risk.

Prescription and Over-the-Counter Drugs

Women may or may not know about pharmaceuticals that are teratogenic or potentially teratogenic. A list of all prescription and over-the-counter (OTC) drugs, as well as homeopathic medicines or vitamins sold by independent dealers, should be obtained. Lithium and isotretinoin (Accutane), known teratogens, are used relatively frequently by women of childbearing age. High-dose vitamins are also common, yet many women do not know that vitamin A consumed in amounts greater than 10,000 IU per day has been found to contribute to birth defects (Rothman et al, 1995). Clients should be encouraged to discuss use of all medications and health care products if a pregnancy is planned.

Obstetric History

Because some obstetric complications tend to recur, information should be obtained about all previous pregnancies. Include the number of pregnancies; the gestational age when the pregnancy ended; the type of delivery; length of labor; birth weight when delivery occurred in the second half of pregnancy; the sex of the child or children; complications; current health of the child or children; perception of previous pregnancy, labor, and birth experiences; and the circumstances surrounding any losses. Box 1-1 summarizes the information that is part of the obstetric history.

Early Pregnancy Loss

Early pregnancy loss is common and is usually sporadic. Recurrent early loss, however, may indicate a need to offer clients testing and evaluation that can identify causes such as immunologic factors, uterine abnormalities, genetic abnormalities, and metabolic and endocrinologic disorders.

For example, structural abnormalities in the reproductive tract such as uterine fibroids, a uterine septum, and a bicornuate uterus may not provide enough room for the growing embryo to implant or grow, thus causing an abortion. Abnormal cervical development or trauma to the cervix from gynecologic procedures may render the cervix incapable of supporting the increasing weight of the growing baby. As a result, the "incompetent" (an unfortunate descriptor) cervix dilates, painlessly, in the midtrimester of pregnancy, and the immature fetus is expelled. A procedure in which a suture is placed through the cervix

Box 1-1. Data to be Obtained for the Obstetric History

- Gravida and para (term, preterm, abortions, living)
- Date of each birth (month and year)
- Outcome
    - Gestational age at birth
    - Type of delivery
    - Length of labor
    - Birth weight
    - Gender
    - Complications during pregnancy, at delivery, postpartum; depression during the year after birth
    - Health at present
    - Feelings about previous pregnancies, birth experiences, parenting
- Names and location of children
- Feelings about any perinatal loss (includes miscarriages, elective abortions, midpregnancy losses, perinatal and neonatal deaths, relinquishment for adoption)
- Feelings about other losses in which children were involved such as SIDS, a childhood death, loss of children to a child protection agency

early in pregnancy can sometimes prevent the otherwise inevitable loss of the baby. Some structural abnormalities may be correctable by surgery.

Extensive investigation into the cause of spontaneous abortion is usually withheld until a woman has had three consecutive, spontaneous abortions (two in an older woman, since early pregnancy wastage increases with maternal age and conception occurs less frequently). When the cause of the loss is unknown, genetic counseling may be indicated.

Preterm Birth

Preterm birth can also recur. A history of one preterm birth increases chances for a second preterm birth by as much as 30%. The risk increases as the number of preterm births increases and decreases with the number of term deliveries (American College of Obstetricians and Gynecologists, 1995, #206). As with early pregnancy loss, the causes of preterm birth are often unknown. Uterine malformations and myomata may be involved, as can infection, although the role of the latter is not yet well defined.

Small-for-Gestational Age Babies

A woman who has had a baby that was small-for-gestational-age (SGA) has an increased chance of having another SGA baby. Charts that plot birth weight and gestational age are available to identify the SGA baby. Meanwhile, two weights may be helpful for you to fix in your mind. The first is that healthy babies at 28 weeks weigh about 1000 g (2 lb, 3 oz). The second is that healthy babies at 36 weeks weigh about 2500 g (5 lb, 8 oz). If a woman tells you that she gave birth at 36 weeks to a baby that weighed 4½ lb, you will know that her baby was SGA.

Smoking

In addition to increasing risk for developing cardiovascular disease, obstructive lung disease, and lung cancer, women who smoke while pregnant subject the fetus to decreased uteroplacental perfusion and oxygenation. Babies born to women who smoke more than half a pack of cigarettes per day are likely to weigh less than they would have weighed if the mother had not smoked. In some cases, the effect on the baby is enough to significantly affect birth weight and jeopardize fetal health. Additionally, there are long-term effects on babies born into households where people smoke. An increased incidence in SIDS, meningococcal disease, pneumonia, asthma, bronchitis, colds, and ear infections has been documented. It is easy to see why health care providers place so much emphasis on smoking cessation for pregnant women.

If a woman who smokes is contemplating a pregnancy, ask if she is ready to stop smoking. A methodical plan for supporting her efforts is often helpful. In most cities the American Cancer Society and the American Lung Association maintain lists of classes available nearby.

Alcohol

There are more than 2 million alcoholic women in the United States. Most are of childbearing age. Fetal alcohol syndrome (FAS), a syndrome of abnormal facial features, stunted growth, behavior problems, and varying degrees of intellectual handicap, is the result of excessive alcohol consumption during pregnancy and is the leading cause of congenital mental retardation. As FAS children get older, they are likely to have problems with memory, abstract thinking, judgement, and impulse control. They are easily distracted, hypersensitive to criticism, and find it difficult to follow through with tasks. Psychosocial problems persist into adulthood.

Alcohol Related Neurodevelopmental Disorder (ARND), formerly known as Fetal Alcohol Effects (FAE), although not a medical diagnosis, refers to children who exhibit the neuropsychological problems of FAS children but lack the facial features. Problems common to children with this disorder may not become obvious until the school years or even later when job difficulties and encounters with the legal establishment are frequent.

The amount and duration of intrauterine exposure to alcohol required to produce these effects is unknown, although a dose–response relationship generally occurs. Greater exposure is associated with more serious effects (Streissguth, 1989). Individual differences in maternal metabolism of alcohol may account for the large number of babies whose mothers drink heavily in pregnancy but escape the syndrome. The number of drinks consumed, exposure during a period of organogenesis, and genetic sensitivity may also play a role. Pregnant women who drink at least one or more drinks per day have a twofold increase in spontaneous abortions (Harlap & Shiono, 1980) and for every two drinks consumed daily in late pregnancy, infant birth weight has been found to be decreased by 160 g (Little, 1977).

Questions about alcohol use can be introduced at any appropriate time during the preconception interview. Sometimes an opening occurs after the clinician asks about parental use of alcohol and drugs. You might say "Could you tell me a little bit about your own experience with alcohol?" and follow with "How old were you when you first tasted something alcoholic? When you started serious drinking? How much are you drinking now?"

No agreed-on definition of alcoholism is in use at the present time. However, two guidelines are: 12 or more drinks per week, or the number of drinks it takes before a woman feels high (8 oz of beer equals 5 oz of wine equals 1½ oz 80-proof alcohol). A woman who states that it takes three or more drinks before she feels the effect might be a problem drinker, since most women feel the effects of alcohol by the second drink.

If you suspect that the client drinks too much, ask "Do you think you have a drinking problem?" ("Drinking problem" may be better understood and accepted than "alcoholism".) If the client does not feel that a problem exists, ask "What would it take for you to think you had a problem?" This question can identify beliefs that interfere with recognition of a personal problem with alcohol.

For example, a woman who was 5 months' pregnant and worked the evening shift drank 40 ounces of beer each night when she arrived home from work. She felt she needed the beer to help her "wind down" enough to sleep. She did not feel that she had a drinking problem. When asked what it would take for her to feel she had a problem, she replied "Drinking all day like my sister does."

Clinicians are often reluctant to question women about their use of alcohol for fear of offending them. The critical nature of this information, however, demands that it be obtained. Establishing a good relationship with the client and finding the right way to introduce the subject are key factors. At times, it may be helpful to approach this topic peripherally. Asking "How has alcohol affected your life in the past?" allows the client to talk about growing up in an alcoholic family and her own use, as well as recent or current use by significant people in her life.

Be sure to ask about the partner's alcohol consumption. A high alcohol intake increases the likelihood of abuse and the use of illicit drugs. Box 1-2 lists additional questions to ask as indicated.

Box 1-2. Questions to Ask About Alcohol Use

1. How has alcohol affected your life in the past? How about now?
2. How often do you have a drink of beer, wine, a wine cooler, hard liquor, or anything containing alcohol?
3. When you drink, how often do you have 1 or 2 drinks? 3 or 4 drinks? go on binges? You could also ask "How much alcohol do you drink a week? a month? a day?" Offer specific choices—a 6-pack, a case?
4. How many drinks does it take to make you feel high?
5. How old were you when you started drinking? When you first got drunk?
6. Has anyone ever expressed concern to you about your drinking?
7. Has your drinking ever led to problems between you and your family?
8. Have you ever been in trouble with the law because of your drinking? Ever been arrested for driving under the influence of alcohol (DUI)? How many times?
9. Do others encourage you to drink?
10. How many close friends or family members drink a lot or have a drinking problem?

13

Illicit and Recreational Drugs

The use of illicit and recreational drugs is widespread. The true extent of use is unknown because the illegal status of these drugs makes users reluctant to discuss them, and the environment in which drug use takes place is often inaccessible to researchers. It is known, however, that neither socioeconomic status nor race and ethnicity predict which women will have a positive result on a toxicologic urine study (Chasnoff, Landress, & Barrett, 1990). Most drug users use more than one drug, and almost all use alcohol as well.

Cocaine affects the part of the brain that regulates feelings of pleasure. It blocks the reabsorption of dopamine, causing neural impulses to keep firing. Pulse and temperature increase, the desire for sex is heightened, and illusions of mental alertness are present. However, euphoria, energy, and the aphrodisiac effect turn into anxiety, exhaustion, and depression. Cocaine is particularly dangerous to the growing fetus. It is associated with spontaneous abortion, preterm delivery, intrauterine growth retardation, and abruptio placenta. One maternal death from vaginal use of cocaine has been reported (Greenland, 1989). For a small number of people who lack an enzyme that breaks cocaine down, one dose of cocaine can kill.

Heroin use is associated with prematurity, intrauterine growth retardation, and withdrawal symptoms in the baby. The effect of marijuana, the most commonly abused illicit drug in this country, is not known, nor is the effect of LSD or amphetamines. A new amphetamine, methcathinone ("cat" on the streets), has spread from labs in Michigan and Wisconsin. It is a synthetic version of cathinone, the active ingredient of the Khat bush found in East Africa, Somalia, Yemen, and the Arabian peninsula. Methcathinone is a highly addictive drug, with twice the stimulus effect of cocaine. Initially, it produces hyperactivity, agitation, and euphoria. It may also induce psychosis, bradycardia, and hypotension (Addiction Counseling Certification Board of Oregon, 1995).

Women who use injectable drugs are at increased risk for AIDS if they share needles, use a drug like cocaine that increases the likelihood of indiscriminate and unprotected sexual activity, or trade sex for drugs. AIDS cases in individuals injecting drugs increased from 17% during 1982 to 1987, to 27% during 1993 to October 1995 (CDC, 1995a).

Determining whether or not a client is using drugs and the extent of use can be difficult. Some clinicians feel it is important to *assume* that a client is using them. These clinicians will ask "What recreational drugs do you use? How much? How many times a day? a week? a month?" "When was the last time you used?"

Other clinicians prefer to ask a general question, such as "Have you ever used recreational drugs—marijuana, cocaine, acid, speed, something similar?" Be sure to specifically mention marijuana because some people do not consider it an illicit or recreational drug. Box 1-3 lists additional questions to ask as appropriate.

Clinicians should know common words for illicit drugs and how these drugs get into the body. For example, methamphetamine is also known as speed, crystal, crank, go, and ice. It can be snorted, injected, smoked, or taken orally (CDC, 1995b).

In some instances, clients are more likely to divulge drug use on a form rather than in a person-to-person interview. Consequently, some offices/clinics have a drug-use form that clients are asked to fill out. Appendix B contains examples of questions about drug use.

Box 1-3. Questions to Ask About Use of Illicit and Recreational Drugs

1. What drugs have you used?
2. Have you ever been a regular user? For how many months or years?
3. When was the last time you used . . . ?
4. How much did you use?
5. Have you also used . . . ?
6. How much of that did you use?
7. What about . . . ?
8. Have you ever been in a drug treatment program? How many times?
9. Have you ever lost a job or been in trouble with the law because of drugs?
10. Have you ever shared needles for drugs?

Environmental Exposures

Exposure to toxic elements in the environment can occur while at work, at home, or at play. While appropriate use of most chemicals is not known to be harmful to the unborn fetus, women should be encouraged to eliminate chemicals or observe appropriate precautions when they are used. Known exposure to harmful agents should be documented. All clients should be asked about current and past exposure to biologic agents, radiation, metals, dust or fibers, fumes, pesticides, and chemicals. Unfortunately, except for higher incidences of cancer, little is known about the effect of these substances on humans.

Clients may or may not be aware of radiation exposure. For example, between 1944 and 1972, more than 2 million people were exposed to radioactive materials released into the air and the Columbia River in southeastern Washington state by the Hanford Project, a federal government project that produced plutonium for nuclear weapons. An individual's dose depended on his or her distance and direction from the site; age during exposure; length of exposure; the amount and source of milk, fresh fruit, and leafy vegetables eaten; the amount and kind of Columbia River fish eaten and where they were caught; and exposure to the river water from jobs, recreation, and irrigation (Oregon Health Division, 1996).

Health care providers need to know when their clients have lived in areas such as Hanford. Information specific to the site may be available to both client and provider. For example, the Hanford Health Education Network has a number of reports available, as well as screening guidelines for thyroid disease. Thyroid problems have been the most common medical problem associated with living near the Hanford site. Appendix C contains a sample exposure history that may be helpful if toxic exposure is suspected.

Psychosocial History

"Hard" data on the role of social and emotional factors on the outcome of pregnancy is difficult to find. Part of the problem is that many factors may be involved, and isolating one or two is impossible. Experienced and caring clinicians, nevertheless, *know* that poverty, inadequate housing, problems with relationships, depression, poor self-esteem, low levels of education, stress, and meager systems of social support put pregnant women at risk. The preconception counseling visit can be used to help mothers assess their psychosocial readiness for parenting. One of the topics that should be discussed is abuse.

History of Abuse

Physical, emotional, and sexual abuse are horrendous crimes which have been committed against women for thousands of years. Society has ignored this abuse for almost as long as the abuse has existed. It is appropriate to ask about a history of abuse at a preconception visit so that women who are presently in an abusive relationship can be offered help and become aware of the likelihood of the abuse increasing during pregnancy.

Women who have been sexually abused in the past can be made aware that memories of the abuse may surface during pregnancy or labor, causing feelings of anxiety, confusion, or sadness. Evolving data suggest that a history of sexual abuse may influence a woman's ability to deliver vaginally. Powerful emotional forces may make women able to "shut labor down" so that they do not have to deal with many people looking at their genitalia or feel the baby emerge from a place that is associated with pain, embarrassment, guilt, and humiliation.

> *The fear of losing control makes some laboring women with a history of sexual abuse struggle against their contractions. Relaxation may be impossible and suggestions from well-meaning childbirth educators or staff to "relax," "surrender," "yield," or "open up," may remind the survivor of the times when she was made to do these things and was hurt. Other suggestions, meant to reassure, such as "trust your body," "Do what your body tells you to do," are incomprehensible to the survivor whose body has been a source of anguish and betrayal. Her efforts to keep labor under her control may actually slow or stop progress (Simkin, 1994).*

While it is not always appropriate to discuss these possibilities at the preconception visit, clinicians should think about follow-up that might be indicated.

It is usually best to ask questions about abuse when alone with the client. If an abusive partner is aware that questions about abuse are being asked, the client may not be allowed to return and continue her care with you. If the client is accompanied by a partner, at the end of the interview you might say "I always like to spend a little time alone with each of the potential parents. Would you excuse us for just a few minutes?" When alone, ask the client if there is any information she would like to share in private. After she responds, tell her that you would like to ask her a few personal questions, questions that are asked of everyone who comes for care. You can add "You don't have to answer any question that you feel is intrusive or none of my business."

A client may or may not wish to admit to an abusive relationship. Incest is particularly difficult to acknowledge because of its profound negative connotations. Clinicians can be helpful by deciding not to ignore the possibility of abuse in any woman's life. The role of the health care provider is to:

Provide a private place to ask questions.
Communicate a willingness to talk about abuse and hear painful information.
Convey to the expectant mother that she is believed, that she was not deserving of the abuse, and that no one has the right to abuse her.
Help her decide if she is safe.
Help her prepare an "action plan" if safety is an issue.

Provide information about community resources.

Initiate a referral if appropriate.

Respect her decision regardless of what it is.

Box 1-4 lists questions that may be appropriate to ask. This list of questions will not be suitable in all situations, nor will the approach and phrasing of the questions fit every clinician's style. Develop a personal list of questions or modify those suggested as you gain experience and as you listen to the way colleagues approach this subject.

If a woman reports having been abused, ask if she has ever talked about the abuse with anyone. Does she have someone whom she talks with now? A woman in a relationship that is currently abusive should be asked if she is in immediate danger. Does she fear for her life? Is there a gun in the house? Are the children in jeopardy? Has she ever thought of leaving her partner because of the abuse?

When appropriate, encourage an "action plan" for leaving. The plan should include a change of clothes for the mother and the children left in a safe place, perhaps with a neighbor or at work; cash for a taxi and quarters for phone calls; car and house keys; a list of emergency phone numbers; important documents such as personal photographs, rent receipts, bank statements, Medicaid certification, a driver's license, birth certificates, and immunization records so that the children can enroll in school; and a safe place to go. It may be appropriate for the

---

Box 1-4. Questions to Ask About Abuse

1. Does your partner ever do anything that scares you? Are you ever frightened by your partner's temper?

2. Have you ever been called names, put down, or unfairly accused?

3. Have you ever been in a relationship where you were pushed, shoved, slapped, hit, punched, kicked, had something thrown at you, or were hurt in any way?

4. Do you ever "give in" because you are afraid of your partner's reaction?

5. Does your partner ever withhold affection as punishment?

6. Does your partner ever threaten to withhold money? Have an affair?

7. Do you ever apologize to others for your partner's behavior?

8. Has your partner ever tried to stop you from seeing friends?

9. Do you feel isolated?

10. Is your partner jealous of your friends?

11. Do you need your partner's permission to do anything?

12. Are you afraid of what will happen next or that you can't survive alone?

13. Do you think your partner is capable of killing you?

14. Do you believe accusations of being stupid, worthless, not doing things right?

(From Slaughter, R., & Kanter, L. (1993). Women being alive. *Domestic Violence: Is It Happening to You?*)

15. How many times in the last year have you been involved in yelling or screaming fights?

16. How many times in the past year have you been hit or had something thrown at you? Do you ever hit back? Ever hit first?

clinician to make the initial contact with a domestic violence shelter or other safe place. A list of names and phone numbers should be available. Many clinics and offices place cards with a list of shelters and emergency phone numbers in the women's restroom.

Some women in abusive situations or with a history of abuse appreciate suggestions of books to read as well as a list of support groups. Lists of these should be available. Appendix D contains a list of references that might be useful. Be certain to read these books yourself before recommending them. When you find a book you like, call your local library to see if the book is one that circulates in the library system. If not, ask for the procedure for recommending new books.

You should also be familiar with counselors, support groups, and other organizations in your area with expertise in counseling women who have been abused. Keep a list with the names, addresses, and phone numbers of these counselors, as well as their fees. Be sure to identify those who use a sliding scale. Make lists also of shelters and support groups. Keep small cards containing this information in the rest room so that women can slip one into a purse. Perhaps most important is realizing that "Simply asking about abuse—and then listening to a patient's story—can be as important as providing resources and physical care" (Titus, 1996).

At some point in the interview with women who have been or who are in an intimate relationship that involves violent or controlling behavior, determine whether or not children in the family have observed the behavior.

The deleterious effects on children who witness physical violence between their parents or caregivers has been well documented. Therefore, if children are living with the client, it is important to ask if the children have seen or heard threats or assaults or have been threatened or assaulted themselves by the abuser (Alpert, 1995).

Discussion of painful issues can be difficult for both clinician and client. Some practitioners hesitate to ask about abuse because they feel they are being intrusive, fear being overwhelmed by the stories, find the stories too painful, think it will take too much time, feel the information is irrelevant, or were taught they should not ask about things they can do nothing about. Some have misperceptions about which women are abused. A personal history of abuse may arouse feelings of anxiety. When this happens, the clinician may find it helpful to work with a counselor or another supportive person until it is possible to be a helpful listener. In the interim, working with a colleague who can elicit the needed information and act in a therapeutic manner may be necessary.

When possible, find an opportunity to speak in private with the woman's partner, asking if there is anything this person wishes to share, something that may or may not relate to pregnancy or parenting. Male partners often have long histories of physical and emotional abuse. Some have been sexually abused as well. If the partner reports a family history of drug or alcohol abuse, ask what that was like as a child. Great pain may have occurred. Sometimes a referral for counseling is appropriate and welcome. Box 1-5 summarizes the information to be obtained at the preconception interview.

Referrals

Information obtained from the history may indicate the need for a referral to community resources for a variety of reasons. Lists containing the following may be appropriate.

- Counseling and mental health centers, their fees, and qualifications of the counselors

Box 1-5. Information to Be Obtained at a Preconception Interview

Genetic background
   Maternal age
   Family history
      Medical history (organic disease, psychiatric diagnoses)
      Ethnic background
      Obstetric history (stillbirth, neonatal death, early SIDS, congenital anomaly including neural tube defect, unusual facial features, genetic or chromosomal disorders, mental retardation, person with three or more spontaneous abortions, client's mother's use of DES, mother or sister(s) with severe preeclampsia)
      Father of the baby and his family (mental retardation or developmental delay, birth defect, unusual facial features, genetic or chromosomal disorder, family member with three or more spontaneous abortions
   Consanguinity (with partner only)
Medical history
Prescription drugs, over-the-counter medicine, herbal remedies, and nutritional supplements
Obstetric history
Smoking
Alcohol
Drugs
Environmental exposures
   Job
   Hobbies
   Geographic location
Abuse
   Physical
   Emotional
   Sexual
Tests to consider
   CBC, rubella titre, varicella titre, HIV, syphilis, hepatitis B, PPD, gonorrhea, chlamydia

- Childbirth classes, the philosophy of the instructor, number of classes in a series, cost, where held, and when
- Stop-smoking programs and their cost
- Alcohol and drug treatment programs, type and length of program, philosophy, and cost
- Parenting classes and their cost
- Immunization clinics and their fees

▼ Laboratory Testing

The approximate cost of testing that might be unique to a given pregnancy such as amniocentesis or blood work should be discussed. Financial support from organizations such as the March of Dimes is sometimes available.

Tests to Validate Maternal Health

Tests to validate maternal health and readiness for pregnancy might include the following:

Complete Blood Count

A complete blood count (CBC) includes numeric counts of the red blood cells (RBCs), white blood cells (WBCs), and platelets; the hemoglobin and hematocrit, and red blood cell indices. The indices refer to three measurements (mean corpuscular volume, MCV; mean corpuscular hemoglobin, MCH; and mean corpuscular hemoglobin concentration, MCHC) that assist in classifying anemias. Box 1-6 identifies normal values for RBC indices. In some laboratories, a CBC also includes a differential white count ("diff"). A CBC is useful in women hoping to conceive because it can lead to early identification of anemia. The algorithm in Figure 1-1 shows how the MCV can be used to identify thalassemia syndromes that can significantly affect perinatal morbidity and mortality. It should be followed when the client is from a group at risk for one of the thalassemias (see page 4).

Rubella Titre

This titre identifies women who have antibodies against rubella. Women without sufficient antibodies are termed "nonimmune" and should be advised to be immunized so that they will not become infected with rubella in early pregnancy, when severe sequelae may result should the fetus become infected. Immunity exists when the rubella titre is more than 1:10. Maternal rubella infection in the first trimester of pregnancy frequently causes congenital rubella syndrome.

Varicella Titre

Varicella during pregnancy can be dangerous for both mother and baby. Maternal disease in the first half of pregnancy may affect the fetus in a variety of ways: deafness, cataracts, chorioretinitis, microcephaly, limb hypoplasia, and skin scarring. After 20 weeks' gestation, maternal varicella may result in blood, liver, and spleen involvement. A pregnant woman with varicella may deliver prematurely and/or develop varicella pneumonia, a serious and often life-threatening disease (Katz et al, 1995). Even in the presence of full pulmonary support, if he-

---

Box 1-6. Normal Values for Red Blood Cell Indices*

Mean Corpuscular Volume (MCV), a measurement of the average size of the RBC: 80–95 fL

Mean Corpuscular Hemoglobin (MCH), a reflection of the amount of hemoglobin per cell: 26–34 pg

Mean Corpuscular Hemoglobin Concentration (MCHC), a measurement of the mean total content of total hemoglobin: 31–36 g/dL

---

* Values vary according to laboratory.

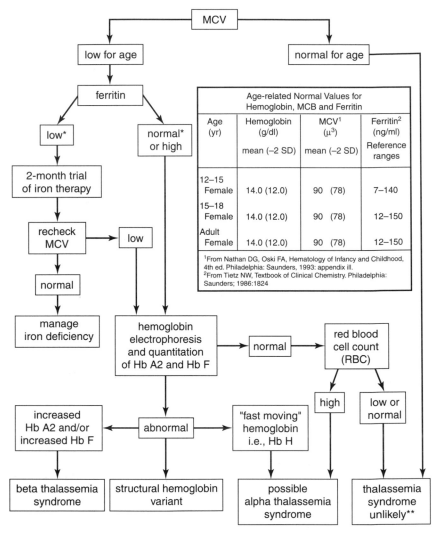

FIGURE 1-1. Algorithm for the detection of thalassemia syndromes using mean corpuscular volume (MCV). (Excluding pregnant women and children less than one year of age.) *From Dumars, K. W., Boehm, C., Eckman, J. R., Giardina, P. J., Lane, P. A., & Shafer, F. E. for the Council of Regional Networks for Genetic Services (CORN). (1996). Practical guide to the diagnosis of thalassemia. *American Journal of Medical Genetics, 62,* p. 31.

moptysis occurs, the maternal death rate can be as high as 50%. If maternal infection occurs around the time of delivery, after the mother has become infected but before she has had time to mount an antibody response, the baby will receive a high viral load. The mortality rate may be as high as 40%.

The recent availability of a varicella vaccine makes it important to determine whether or not a woman anticipating a pregnancy is protected. A woman who knows she has had varicella in the past can be assumed to be immune. Women who do not know if they have had varicella should be encouraged to have a titre drawn and vaccine administered before conception if protection is not demonstrated.

Human Immunodeficiency Virus (HIV)

Whether or not HIV disease is affected by pregnancy is not known. It is known, however, that the virus can be passed from the mother to her baby. While at one time it was thought that perinatal transmission might be as high as 50%, current research suggests that it is 15% to 30%. A recently published study involving HIV-infected women in Boston, Chicago, Manhattan, Brooklyn, San Juan, and Houston found a transmission rate of 17.7% among infants followed for at least 6 months (Sheon et al, 1996).

Women who are HIV-positive and contemplate a pregnancy often benefit from meeting with clinicians and mental health counselors who have experience caring for HIV-positive pregnant women. Decisions about pregnancy in these instances are highly personal and complex.

Syphilis

Maternal syphilis can cause prematurity, stillbirth, and congenital malformations. The fetus is vulnerable throughout pregnancy, and attack rates are highest in cases of primary or secondary disease. *Adequate treatment* of syphilis before conception removes risk to the fetus.

Hepatitis B Surface Antigen

Pregnancy rarely alters the course of hepatitis B infection. The concern when a pregnant woman has this disease is that the baby will become infected at delivery and die of hepatocellular carcinoma or cirrhosis, or become a chronic carrier at risk for transmitting the disease to others. Identification of women who are chronic carriers of hepatitis B is important so that they can access medical care and make good decisions about a future pregnancy. A positive hepatitis B surface antigen documents a need for additional testing. The tests performed vary from institution to institution.

PPD (Tuberculosis)

Women who are in high-risk groups for tuberculosis (Box 1-7) should be offered PPD testing.

Tests for Chlamydia and Gonorrhea

While tests for chlamydia and gonorrhea are usually part of an initial prenatal examination, women who have a history of multiple sexual partners or who have a partner who has had other partners should be offered testing if pregnancy is desired. Both gonorrhea and chlamydia can cause infertility.

Box 1-7. Women At Risk for Tuberculosis

- Low income and medically underserved
- From countries where TB is endemic
- Intravenous drug users
- Health care workers
- Residents of extended care facilities or other institutions, including jails

From Leiner, S., & Mays, M. (1996). Diagnosing latent and active pulmonary tuberculosis: A review for clinicians. *Nurse Practitioner, 21*(2), pp. 91–92.

Genetic Counseling

Box 1-8 lists the conditions and situations in which a referral for genetic counseling is usually appropriate. Genetic counseling involves a meeting between the client and a specially trained person to thoroughly review the client's personal and family medical history. Medical records may be reviewed and, at times, a physical examination will be performed. On the basis of this information, additional laboratory tests and clinical evaluations from medical specialists such as gynecologists, neurologists, and ophthalmologists may be requested.

When a genetic problem is identified, counseling would include a discussion of the diagnosis, prognosis, recurrence risks, course of the disease, treatment options, and medical and social support services available. Women referred because of maternal age would have an opportunity to discuss the incidence of chromosomal abnormalities in their age group and would be apprised of the benefits and risks of diagnostic procedures.

Women whose babies have been exposed to a teratogen can also benefit from genetic counseling, since most genetic counseling services have incorporated this component into the counseling they provide. A genetic consultation is probably not necessary when the baby's father was exposed to a teratogen; the family history includes only one case of a generally noninherited condition such as cerebral palsy; or when the family history includes a single distant relative (great-aunts and great-uncles, cousins) with a multifactorial condition (cleft lip or palate, clubfoot, multiple sclerosis) other than neural tube defects or congenital heart disease.

A sickle cell screen should be offered to those of African descent to test for sickle cell disease, and Ashkenazi Jews and French Canadians should be offered testing for Tay-Sachs disease.

▼ Health Education

Options for Birth Attendant and Place of Birth

Women or couples planning a pregnancy may or may not know that there are major differences in philosophy about prenatal care and birth. These differences often depend on the education and experience of the health care provider. For example, certified nurse-midwives, direct-entry midwives, family practice physicians, naturopaths, and obstetricians all provide prenatal care and assist at

---

Box 1-8. Conditions or Situations in Which Genetic Counseling is Appropriate

Conditions or situations in either parent or their family

1. Possible carrier status for a genetic disease such as sickle cell (of African heritage), Tay-Sachs disease (Ashkenazi Jewish and French Canadian heritage), thalassemias (North, West, and Central Africa, Italy, Sicily, Greece, the Middle East, South Asia, Southeast Asia, Southern China, Pacific Islands)
2. Adult-onset disability of genetic origin
3. Behavioral disorders of genetic origin
4. Down syndrome or other chromosomal abnormality
5. A family history of a known genetic disorder
6. Mental retardation or developmental delay
7. Chronic neurologic or neuromuscular childhood disorders
8. Short stature and other growth disorders
9. Infertility or sterility
10. Exposure to potentially mutagenic or teratogenic agents
11. Multiple family members with the same condition even when it is not thought to be genetic

Conditions or situations in the mother

12. Has had 3 or more unexplained, consecutive, spontaneous first trimester losses or 2 or more spontaneous first trimester losses if she is over 30 years of age
13. Is aged 35 or older
14. Has had a previous infant with a birth defect when no cytogenic study was performed (single anomalies, multiple defects, metabolic disorders)
15. Has had a neonatal death or an unexplained stillborn baby
16. Has had a baby die with a case of atypical SIDS (death before 1 month of age or after 12 months)
17. Has a risk because of consanguinity

Conditions or situations in the father

18. Has been the father in three consecutive first trimester losses

---

birth, but the manner in which each goes about doing this work is highly variable. Learn about the practitioners in your community, the birth centers, the hospitals, their policies, their costs, the availability of home birth. Offer clients a list of questions that might be asked of potential providers so that an informed choice about both provider and place of birth can be made. Participants in a health care plan should be encouraged to study the provisions of the plan to see what is covered.

At the preconception visit, determine whether or not the woman or couple know about options for birth attendant and place of birth. What is important during the pregnancy? What would make them feel like they are getting good care? Have they thought about what might be important in labor, at the birth, immediately after the birth?

Some newspapers publish a yearly update on birthing services in the community. When this happens, save the report to share with people looking for this information. If this information is not currently available in your community, consider gathering it. The Missouri Department of Health has published "Buyer's Guide: Obstetrical Services" (1994), a 21-page booklet reporting on selected quality-of-care indicators for hospitals in St. Louis and eastern Missouri. Copies can be obtained for $3 from Box 570, Jefferson City, MO, 65102, (314-751-6279). This kind of information can give consumers important information about community hospitals. Similar information about birth centers and home birth services may be available in some communities.

Recommendations for Clients

General information that clinicians can give to women wishing to conceive might include the following items. If you provide these recommendations in writing, adjust the wording to fit your client population.

Realize that there probably isn't one food pyramid that fits everyone. Asian diets rely on an abundance of plant foods. Some feel that the United States Department of Agriculture (USDA) pyramid, which treats animal and vegetable protein the same, may promote disease rather than confer benefits. Appendix E provides a guide to daily food choices and charts that can be helpful for nutrition counseling.

1. Keep a menstrual history calendar so that the first day of your last normal menstrual period will be known. A menstrual history gives the clinician an opportunity to provide information about the fertile period and to identify irregularities that might indicate problems that could preclude or delay conception. Intermenstrual bleeding not related to a contraceptive method should be investigated.

2. Time intercourse to coincide with new research that indicates a woman's fertile period begins 4 to 5 days before ovulation.

3. If stopping the birth control pill to get pregnant, stop the pill at the end of a pill package. Wait until you have one menstrual period on your own before trying to conceive. Do not count the period you will have during the last week of your 28-day pill pack. Use a barrier method of contraception in the interim. (A small number of women who stop using the oral contraceptive will have a post–pill amenorrhea for up to 6 months. When this happens, the date of conception in a pill user who has not menstruated will be unknown and an accurate "due date" will be difficult to determine.

   Certain contraceptive methods may influence the time frame within which conception occurs. For example, women who are using depot-medroxyprogesterone acetate (DMPA) for contraception should know that it may take up to 24 months for conception to occur after discontinuing this method. However, almost 70% of women using DMPA will have conceived within 12 months following discontinuation.

4. Eat a well-balanced diet with appropriately sized portions. Keep caffeine-containing beverages to two per day, recognizing that no one really knows how much caffeine per day might be harmful.

   Guidelines for the professional or elite athlete should be individualized. Diets of these women may not be nutritionally sound, particularly in calories, and they may consume large quantities of vitamins which could be teratogenic. Athletes in the professional or elite category should discuss their training and competition programs with a perinatologist.

5. Be aware that folic acid, an essential B vitamin, can reduce the risk of having a baby with neural tube defects (NTDs) (anencephaly, spina bifida, meningomyelocele). Take a prenatal vitamin, a multivitamin containing 400 μg (0.4 mg) of the B vitamin folic acid or, preferably, just 400 μg of folic acid from 4 weeks before conception through the first month of pregnancy to decrease the likelihood of having a baby with an NTD. Folic acid tablets will be considerably less expensive than prenatal vitamins, even the generic brands. Many nonprescription brands of multivitamins, including Centrum, Stresstabs, Theragran, Unicap, Femiron, and Myadec, contain sufficient folic acid. Folic acid dosage in prenatal vitamins varies. If you have been advised to take 4 *mg* daily, do **not** take 4 multivitamins each day as dangerous levels of vitamins A and D can increase the risk of other birth defects. Instead, take 4 tablets containing 1 mg of folic acid or 3 tablets containing 1 mg of folic acid plus 1 prenatal multivitamin containing the higher dose of 1 mg of folic acid.

(Since more than half of all pregnancies in the United States are unplanned, and since most women in this country consume only half of the recommended amount of folic acid, this recommendation from the Centers for Disease Control applies to all women of childbearing age who could become pregnant. While it is possible to get enough folic acid from dietary sources, less than 20% of the population gets 0.4 mg or more from eating (Niebyl, 1995, p. 49). Food sources high in folic acid include green vegetables, legumes, dried beans, egg yolks, beets, whole wheat bread, liver, fortified breakfast cereals, and citrus fruits and juices (Niebyl, 1995, p. 46).

Women who have had a previous baby with an NTD or a family history of an NTD should take 4 *mg* daily. Also at increased risk for NTDs are women with diabetes and women with a history of seizures. They should also take 4 *mg* per day to bring their risk down to that of the general population.

6. When supplementary vitamins are consumed, keep the vitamin A intake below 8000 IU daily to avoid the possibility of a teratogenic effect from a high vitamin A intake (Murphy, P).

7. Avoid cigarettes. This includes marijuana. Cigarette smoking in amounts greater than half a pack per day lowers birth weight—approximately 1 lb for every pack smoked. After the baby is born, secondhand smoke will increase the incidence of ear and upper respiratory infections and asthma. Ask your partner to stop smoking also.

8. Avoid alcoholic beverages. This includes beer, wine, wine coolers, hard liquor, and cough and cold medicines that contain alcohol.

9. Avoid illicit and recreational drugs. This includes marijuana.

10. Avoid over-the-counter, prescription, and homeopathic medicines until their use is discussed with the health care provider. Use acetaminophen for pain relief and fever reduction rather than aspirin or a nonsteroidal antiinflammatory agent (NSAID) such as Advil.

11. Be certain that adequate protection of pelvic structures occurs if an x-ray film is necessary.

12. Try to exercise for 20 to 30 minutes at least 4 times a week.
    (A small study from Sweden of women with back and posterior pelvic pain reported: "An interesting finding not related to our program was the effect of physical fitness exercise before pregnancy, which reduced the risk of developing back pain in pregnancy." Unfortunately, the authors did not describe any fitness program (Ostgaard, 1994).

13. Be aware of environmental toxins. Toxicants in the home environment include indoor air pollution (tobacco smoke, wood stoves, gas ranges, building materials such as formaldehyde and asbestos); household cleaners, glues, lead paint, and paint stripper; pesticides and lawn care products; a tainted water supply, and contaminated soil.

14. If you have not had chicken pox, get the vaccine or have a blood test to see if you are already protected, then avoid pregnancy for 3 months. Chicken pox infection during pregnancy is associated with significant problems for both mother and baby.

15. Be sure your immunizations are up-to-date. Booster doses of tetanus-diphtheria toxoid (Td) are recommended every 10 years unless you are injured and have a tetanus-prone wound. In these cases a booster dose is given after 5 years. The vaccine is 99% effective (CDC, 1993, "Reported vaccine-preventable diseases.")

16. Congenital toxoplasmosis, although rare, can occur when women acquire the infection while pregnant. If you have a cat, decide on what precautions you will take in regard to who will change the litter box, what protective material will be worn while changing it (if you will be changing it), and how often the litter will be changed. Ideally, a non-pregnant person should change the litter box. If this is not possible, change the litter box daily. Wear protective gloves. A mask is probably not necessary while changing the litter box because infection by inhalation is rare. Wear gloves when gardening because cat feces may be in the soil. Do not allow cats outside where they might attack and eat an infected mouse. Bear in mind, however, that few cats, even those that are strays, are infected with toxoplasmosis. Stray cats should not be allowed in the house, and handwashing should occur after pregnant women have handled a cat but especially before eating (Gibbs & Sweet, 1994).

    In most instances, women can be reassured that their likelihood of acquiring a primary toxoplasmosis infection in pregnancy is small unless they have had direct contact with cat feces that are 4 days old. It takes this long for the oocysts in the feces to become infective.

17. Avoid undercooked meat, as it is a potential source of toxoplasmosis.

18. If there are pets in the home, such as ferrets and some breeds of dogs, that could be dangerous to babies or children, consider finding other homes for these animals. If sanitation is a problem because of many pets or animals in the house, consider finding new homes for these animals, or learn and observe appropriate hygienic procedures.

19. While precise data on the timing and amount of heat exposure necessary to cause congenital anomalies is not available, sufficient concern exists to recommend avoiding saunas throughout pregnancy. Also avoid hot tubs with a temperature above 100.4°F, particularly in the first third of pregnancy.

20. Wear seat belts with both shoulder and lap belts. The lower strap should be placed as snug as is comfortable below your abdomen. Position the shoulder belt above your uterus. Make sure the headrest is at a height to protect your head from whiplash (Schoenfeld et al, 1987).

Many women and couples will appreciate a list of books to read before and during pregnancy. Visit your public libraries and local book stores to see what is available. Prepare an annotated bibliography listing your favorite references. Stores like Goodwill and Salvation Army often carry used books at affordable prices. Your clinic or office may be willing to purchase these to lend to clients.

▼ Conclusion

While preconception counseling is not a frequent occurrence in the United States, all clinicians who care for women in the childbearing years should be prepared to ask the questions and provide the advice required by this kind of meeting. The issues raised are different from those encountered during a prenatal visit, and clinicians must be aware of the special concerns that should be addressed.

The Initial
Prenatal Visit

▼ Definitions

In every specialty there is a language through which specialists communicate important information to each other. Box 2-1 identifies some of the terms used in obstetrics that describe a woman in relation to pregnancy.

The outcomes of a woman's pregnancies are commonly summarized by a 4-digit designation following the word *para.* The first digit refers to the number of term pregnancies (carried to the end of the 36th week), the second to the number of preterm pregnancies (those between 20 and 36 weeks' gestation), the third to the number of abortions (spontaneous and elective as well as ectopic pregnancies) through the 19th week of gestation, and the fourth to the number of living children. Remembering the mnemonic, **T**ennessee **P**ower **a**nd **L**ight, may be helpful. (T stands for term, P for preterm, A for abortion, and L for living children.)

The summarization of pregnancy outcomes is prefaced by the word *gravida.* The current pregnancy is included. The final description reads *gravida* followed by the number of times the woman has been pregnant and *para* followed by four numbers, each describing a different aspect of pregnancy outcome. For example, the status of a woman who is pregnant for the third time and has had one first trimester spontaneous abortion and one full-term pregnancy resulting in a living child would be *gravida 3, para 1011 (or G3, P1011).*

▼ The History

Conclusive studies documenting the cause or causes of poor pregnancy outcome are either not yet available, or the complex interplay of multiple factors makes the establishment of causality impossible at this time. Risk assessment

---

Box 2-1. Terms Used to Describe a Woman in Relation to Pregnancy

Gravida: A woman who is or has been pregnant
Nulligravida: A woman who has never been and is not currently pregnant
Primigravida: A woman who is pregnant for the first time
Para: A number that by itself refers to the number of babies delivered that were of sufficient size (500 g) or gestational age (20 wks) to be considered viable *or a series of* numbers that summarize the outcomes of previous pregnancies
Nullipara: A woman in her first pregnancy, as well as a woman who has not carried a pregnancy beyond an elective or spontaneous abortion
Primipara: A woman who has had one pregnancy in which the fetus reached the age of viability
Multipara: A woman who has carried two or more pregnancies (as opposed to fetuses) to viability

From Cunningham, F.G., MacDonald, P.C., Gant, N.F., Leveno, K.J., & Gilstrap, L.C., III. (1993). *Williams obstetrics* (19th ed.). Norwalk, CT: Appleton & Lange, 248–249.

tools used in the past to assign a level of risk to pregnant women in hopes of providing the expertise and supervision appropriate to the level-of-risk status have generally been discarded as they have been shown to be poor predictors of who will have a problem and who will not (Collaborative Group, 1993). Still, certain conditions are known to influence the outcome of pregnancy. A thorough and purposeful history provides the basis for anticipating problems and planning care.

Almost every woman is somewhat nervous at her first prenatal visit. A minute or two of social chitchat often puts the new client at ease unless, of course, it is apparent that she is in either physical or emotional distress. If she is alone when you meet her, you might ask if someone came with her and, if so, whether she would like that person to be with her during the interview or physical examination. Be sure to add, however, that some of the questions you will ask are of a personal nature. Assure her that the questions are asked of each person because they help anticipate problems and identify special tests and procedures that should be done.

A helpful way to establish rapport at the initial prenatal visit is to ask "Is this a good time to be having a baby?" You can rejoice with women who are delighted with their condition and empathize with women who are not. Empathy can be a powerful tool, and listening, by itself, can be therapeutic.

In a prenatal clinic, the reason for the visit is almost always the initiation of prenatal care but might also be to discuss the clinic's philosophy of care, to obtain a referral for genetic counseling, or to consider options in regard to continuing the pregnancy. Once the purpose of the visit is identified, ask if there is anything else the client wants to find out or talk about. Once her questions and concerns are addressed, she is more likely to be able to concentrate on your questions. Keep asking "Anything else?" until she no longer has a question for you.

While every office or clinic has a history form that typically asks for demographic information, menstrual history, contraceptive history, obstetrical history, medical and surgical history, and family history, psychosocial information and health-related practices usually are not emphasized even though that information is essential for good care. Clinicians almost always need to ask additional questions to assure that the data are complete. Begin the initial history by selecting an area in which the questions are not likely to be threatening. Since the client has scheduled this visit because she is pregnant, the menstrual history is usually a safe place to start.

Menstrual History

An accurate picture of the client's menstrual history frequently helps establish estimated date of delivery (EDD), still known as estimated date of confinement (EDC) in some places. The EDD is determined by making an internationally recognized and accepted calculation determined by following Naegele's rule. The calculation adds 9 months and 7 days to the first day of the last normal menstrual period (LNMP) or subtracts 3 months, then adds 7 days and 1 year. For example, if the 1st day of the LNMP was January 10, adding 9 months and 7 days gives a due date of October 17. If the first day of the LNMP was November 18, it is easier to count backwards, so subtract 3 months, then add 7 days and 1 year, for an EDD of August 25. At times you need to move into a new month. Suppose the LNMP was September 26. Counting back 3 months, you get June 26. Now add 7 days and 1 year. You get July 3. (June has only 30 days.)

Drug companies often distribute gestation calculators ("wheels") to use to quickly determine the EDD and gestational age in weeks. Some wheels also note mean fetal weight and length for each gestational week. These calculators should not be used to determine the EDD because the calculator-determined EDD will vary as much as 4 days from the EDD determined by Naegele's rule. While this may seem trivial, extensive testing for fetal well-being often begins at 41½ weeks' gestation, and the EDD identified by a gestation calculator is likely to be earlier than the date arrived at using Naegele's rule, resulting in unnecessary expense and anxiety. Everyone should use the same approach for determining the EDD, and Naegele's rule is the accepted standard. Save the wheel for calculating weeks' gestation, as precision in determining gestational age at an uncomplicated prenatal visit is not as important as precision in determining the due date.

Additional information about the menstrual cycle that should be obtained includes the frequency of menses and the duration of bleeding. When women have menstrual cycles that vary by 7 or more days in either direction from the norm of 28 days, the EDD should be adjusted appropriately. For example, in Naegele's rule a woman with 35-day cycles would have 14 days rather than 7 days added, and a woman with 21-day cycles would have no days added. When a woman's last menstrual period has been shorter or lighter than usual, it may be impossible to know whether or not the woman was already pregnant when the bleeding occurred. If supporting data such as the date of quickening and fetal heart tones heard with a fetoscope are missing or confusing, an ultrasound examination may be required for accurate dating.

▶ **SOMETHING FUN**

> The practice of speaking of pregnancy in terms of weeks of gestation may be confusing to women who are pregnant for the first time. While it is usually not possible to give each expectant mother a gestation calculator, you can place the gestation calculator on a copy machine and make a copy of the wheel to give to the client. Arrange the wheel so that the 40-week mark coincides with the EDD.

Contraceptive History

Obtain a contraceptive history because hormonal contraception may affect the EDD, and because use of other methods may help "date" the pregnancy. When a woman finishes the hormone-containing pills in a package of oral contraceptives, the menstrual period she will subsequently have is termed a "withdrawal bleed." It occurs not because of the woman's natural hormonal influences but because hormonal support of the endometrium supplied by the oral contraceptive has been withdrawn. Spontaneous menstruation may or may not occur at the usual time. Lack of spontaneous menses is called post-pill amenorrhea. It can last some months. Because ovulation can occur before resumption of menses, conception can occur during the period of amenorrhea, making accurate dating of the pregnancy difficult. Women who become pregnant without a spontaneous menstrual period after stopping "the pill" should have a sonogram to accurately determine the EDD. A sonogram for accurate dating is also indicated when pregnancy occurs before resumption of spontaneous menses in association with or after use of other hormonal contraceptive methods (ie, Norplant and Depo-Provera).

On rare occasions pregnancy will occur with an IUD in place. When this occurs, remove the IUD if the strings are visible. This procedure may be done by a nurse practitioner during the first trimester, but is best referred to a physician after the 13th week. Removing the IUD decreases the chances for a miscarriage, and leaving the IUD in place increases the chances for a mid-trimester septic abortion. A history of prior IUD use increases the chances for an ectopic pregnancy.

Obstetric History

Essential information about previous pregnancies includes the month and year that the pregnancy ended, the gestational age at the termination of the pregnancy, the type of delivery (spontaneous, forceps, vacuum extraction, or Cesarean), the length of labor (preferably from the first contraction), birth weight, sex of each child, and any complications. When describing pregnancies that ended before 20 weeks, differentiate between spontaneous, elective, and therapeutic abortions as well as ectopic pregnancy. Additionally, the current physical and emotional health of each child should be noted. Note each child's name in the history. This allows the provider to refer to the children as individuals and is useful in facilitating the client–provider relationship.

Interpregnancy Interval

The month and year of the births are important to determine interpregnancy interval. When data are conflicting, there *may* be a risk for preterm birth when the interval between birth and the next pregnancy in certain populations is less than 12 months. Anemia is more frequent when the interbirth interval is less than 1 year.

Outcome of Pregnancies

Gestational Age

The gestational age at birth of previous babies should be known because preterm birth tends to recur and because some women have trouble bonding with babies who have been hospitalized for a long time. A painless delivery early in the third trimester may indicate an "incompetent" cervix, and repeated early losses may indicate a genetic problem.

Type of Delivery

Note whether previous births were vaginal, Cesarean, or assisted with forceps or a vacuum extractor. If a woman has previously had a Cesarean birth, she may be a candidate for a vaginal birth with the present pregnancy. The decision usually depends on the location of the incision that was made into the uterus, the ability of the hospital birthing unit to respond promptly should uterine rupture occur, and the desires of the expectant mother. If the uterine incision was made low in the uterus and cut horizontally (low transverse Cesarean section) rather than vertically (classic Cesarean section), an attempt can usually be made to deliver the baby vaginally. The direction of the skin incision may or may not reflect the direction of the uterine incision.

Obtain copies of the medical records of both the labor and the surgery, when possible, to document the placement of the uterine scar. Records should also be obtained whenever a birth was assisted with forceps or a vacuum extractor. This facilitates understanding the reason for an instrument delivery and may help the birth attendant avoid problems during labor and birth with the present pregnancy.

Length of Labor

Length of labor is important because a long labor may also reflect a problem that could recur. This is particularly true when long labors are a pattern. A disproportion between the presenting part and the maternal pelvis may have occurred. Fortunately, long first labors are seldom followed by other long labors. It is a good idea, however, to request a copy of the labor and birth record whenever a woman reports a labor longer than 24 hours. Short labors also should be noted, as these often repeat. When the labor was short, clinicians often request that women notify the birth attendant early in labor. Occasionally, induction of labor is appropriate so that the birth can occur under controlled circumstances.

Length of labor may be difficult to determine because clinicians vary in the point they choose for the start of labor. Some choose the very first contraction, some like to select the time at which the contractions became "regular," and some select the point at which they became painful.

Birth Weight

Birth weight is important to identify babies who were small for gestational age (SGA) or large for gestational age (LGA), conditions likely to recur. When a vaginal birth has occurred, birth weight demonstrates that a baby of a certain size successfully traversed the maternal pelvis.

Gender

Discussing the sex of previous babies provides an opportunity for the clinician to ask the client about her feelings about daughters and sons, as the case may be, and her preferences and those of her partner in regard to the sex of the present baby. This knowledge can be useful when the sex of the baby is different from a strongly expressed preference.

Complications

Any complication associated with any pregnancy should be known so that those complications known to repeat can be anticipated. Ectopic pregnancy, for example, tends to recur. Spontaneous abortion due to chromosome and genetic abnormalities and second trimester losses from an incompetent cervix may also recur. Other conditions that tend to recur include congenital anomalies, gestational diabetes, preecclampsia, intrauterine growth retardation, shoulder dystocia, postpartum depression, and postpartum hemorrhage caused by uterine atony. When these conditions are reported, copies of medical records should be obtained whenever possible.

Current Health of Children

The outcome of each pregnancy and the current health status of the children should be noted. Illness, disability, emotional problems, and discipline issues can create great stress in families. Referrals may be indicated. Also ask about the location of each child as the birth mother is not always the custodial parent.

Perception of Previous Pregnancy and Birth Experiences

Ask about the client's perception of previous pregnancies and births. What went well? Was anything awful? What would she like to do differently this time? How does she feel about any anesthesia that was or was not administered? Is there something about which she is fearful? Note in the record what the client says. It may be useful later in pregnancy when discussing feelings about the upcoming labor and birth. Women who have had a traumatic birth experience may benefit from referral to a birth counselor or to a therapist. When help from one of these professionals is not possible, the clinician may be able to arrange extra time to listen, support, and help women prepare for the coming birth.

Loss of a Child

A woman who has had a perinatal loss, whether it was a miscarriage, an elective abortion, a stillbirth, a neonatal death, or relinquishment of a baby for adoption, should be asked how that experience has affected her. What was it like? What got her through it? Does she still think about that baby? Is she still grieving? Was the relationship with her partner strained as a result of the loss? How are things now?

Women who have relinquished a baby can be asked if they often think about the child. Expect tears when you ask this question, as there is often unhealed grief. Don't be afraid to ask, however, as women are usually grateful that someone is willing to acknowledge their continuing pain. Not all women, of course, will feel this way. Some have put their experience in the past and rarely or never return to it. Women who have relinquished a child may be asked if they have thought of "searching" for the child. Women who are themselves adopted can be asked if they think about their birth parents.

Each woman—and many clinicians—differ in their feelings about this process. Often a referral to someone who can help the client think through her feelings and consider the pros and the cons of searching will be appropriate. The International Soundex Reunion Registry (ISSR) gives birth parents and the children they relinquished an opportunity to advise each other of their willingness to be contacted. Clients often appreciate the address of ISRR (see Appendix F).

Women whose children live with another person, whether because of child custody arrangements or loss of the children to a child protective agency, should be given an opportunity to talk about that experience and their feelings about it. Almost all women who have lost a child for whatever reason experience profound grief. Women may or may not have been able to talk about their grief. Often the mere fact that the clinician asks about and is willing to allow grieving mothers a chance to talk about their pain, anger, and disappointment can be therapeutic. A referral to a support group may be helpful.

Medical–Surgical History

Gynecologic History

A history of certain gynecologic conditions is particularly important during pregnancy because of their potential for affecting the outcome of pregnancy. Venereal warts, for example, can occasionally grow so large that a Cesarean birth is required. Pelvic inflammatory disease (PID) is associated with an increase in the risk for ectopic pregnancy, and herpes simplex type II can cause severe neurological damage and even death for the baby. Information about a history of infertility, gonorrhea, chlamydia, syphilis, and abnormal vaginal bleeding, as well as an abnormal Pap smear and the date of the most recent Pap smear, should also be obtained so that a complete gynecologic picture is available.

Human Papilloma Virus (HPV)

HPV is a highly contagious virus that often causes condyloma acuminata, sometimes referred to as venereal warts. The warts can be found on the cervix and the vaginal wall, in the urethra, and on the buttocks, anus, and external genitalia. HPV is the most common viral sexually transmitted disease. In rare instances, babies born to mothers with HPV infection will have respiratory problems since the warts can grow in the respiratory tract and cause recurrent respiratory papillomatosis. Lesions on the vocal chords or in the upper airway can usually be controlled with laser surgery but lesions in the lungs can be fatal.

Women with certain types of HPV have a higher incidence of cervical cancer (HPV types 16,18, 45, and 56) (Ferenczy, 1995). Unfortunately, typing of lesions is not generally available. Therefore, regular Pap smears are particularly important for women with HPV. During pregnancy, venereal warts may be treated weekly with local applications of trichloroacetic acid after protecting surrounding tissue. Podophyllin is contraindicated in pregnancy because it is embryotoxic and teratogenic. Laser therapy, used in nonpregnant women, can lead to severe bleeding in pregnant women. When venereal warts enlarge significantly during pregnancy, look carefully at their point of origin. Although some may appear to obstruct the vaginal opening, they may arise from a single stalk that can easily be pushed aside as the baby's head is born.

Pelvic Inflammatory Disease

A clinician should know about a history of PID as early as possible in pregnancy because a single instance of PID increases a woman's chances of having an ectopic pregnancy sevenfold (Oregon Health Division, 1995). Any instance of cramping or bleeding in women with this history requires an ultrasound examination to verify that the pregnancy is in the uterus.

Herpes

Neonatal herpes infection can cause severe neurologic damage to the baby and neonatal death. Infection occurs when the virus gains entrance to the uterine cavity subsequent to rupture of the membranes or at delivery as the fetus passes through an infected cervix or lower genital tract. The fetus may also become infected in utero when the first episode of genital herpes occurs during pregnancy. Pregnant women should be asked to report all lesions noted during the pregnancy, and a culture should be obtained to confirm the diagnosis if not previously verified.

A pregnant woman who reports a history of herpes or a history of a partner with herpes should be counseled about notifying the clinician as soon as she thinks she is in labor so that an appropriate decision about route of delivery can be made. If prodromal symptoms—often a feeling of numbness or tingling where the external body lesion will appear—or a lesion are present when labor occurs or the membranes rupture, delivery is usually by Cesarean section because of the presence of a high viral load.

Some women may not always be aware of a herpes lesion, even when it is on the vulva. Perineal lesions are particularly likely to go undetected, and cervical lesions generally cause no symptoms. Early in labor a thorough inspection of the external genitalia and a speculum examination of the vagina and cervix should be performed in women with a history of herpes as well as in women who have had a partner with herpes, to identify lesions not readily apparent. In some practices, herpes lesions noted around the anus or other areas somewhat removed from the vulva may be covered with a gauze square during labor and at the time of birth. Whether or not a Cesarean birth is truly indicated at all in the presence of prodromal symptoms or herpes lesions is currently being studied.

Organic Disease

Box 2-2 outlines the questions to ask for this portion of the history. While not every disease entity and disorder will have an effect on or be affected by pregnancy, asking about each is essential to obtaining a complete data base. Women with chronic or debilitating health histories, as well as women with diseases such as chronic hypertension, SLE, insulin-dependent diabetes mellitus, cardiac and pulmonary disease, and certain anemias, among other diseases, should receive their maternity care from an obstetrician or a perinatologist when possible. The dose of maternal thyroid medicine in pregnancy often needs to be increased. A thyroid-stimulating hormone (TSH) level is a good way to screen for this disease. TSH levels should be checked each trimester to see if the medication dosage should be adjusted. All states have mandatory newborn testing for congenital hypothyroidism.

Surgery, Accidents, and Hospitalizations

A thorough history includes information about operations, trauma, emergency room visits, and hospital stays. While some of this data may not relate to pregnancy or birth, important information such as the use of blood products between 1978 and 1985 (when AIDS testing was not conducted) or pelvic trauma may be elicited. A woman who tells of frequent emergency room visits for accidents such as walking into doors or falling down stairs should be asked about abuse.

Psychiatric Problems

It is important to determine whether or not a pregnant woman has had a diagnosed mental illness for three reasons: there may be a genetic component to psychiatric illness, pregnancy may exacerbate the illness, and psychotropic drugs may be contraindicated in pregnancy. Common psychiatric diagnoses include Major Depressive Disorder, Dysthymia, Panic Disorder, and Generalized Anxiety Disorder.

Depression

Depression is a relatively common finding in women. Many women suffer needlessly from it because they do not recognize their symptoms as depression; they feel they should be able to "get through it" by themselves; they do not realize that psychotropic medicine and therapy can help; or they have no money with which to seek professional help. Ask specifically about symptoms of depression. You might start by asking:

Have you ever been depressed?

Have you ever had any emotional or mental problems? A nervous breakdown? ("Nervous breakdown" may be better understood than "mental illness.") If "yes," have you taken any medicine for the problem? Have you ever been hospitalized?

Have you ever had counseling?

Have you ever been suicidal? (Ever tried to kill yourself?) If "yes," ask "Could you tell me a little bit about what was happening in your life when you had counseling?" Then ask "How long did the counseling last? Was it helpful? Have you ever thought about getting more?"

How would you describe your mental health now? (You might ask her to rate her mental health on a scale of 1 to 10, with 1 being "poor" and 10 being "great.")

Box 2-2. Data to be Obtained for the Medical/Surgical History

Medical/Surgical History

1. Headaches
2. Seizures/epilepsy
3. Anemia
4. Asthma
5. Arthritis
6. Diabetes
7. Bronchitis/pneumonia
8. High blood pressure
9. Urinary tract infection
10. Thrombophlebitis
11. Varicose veins
12. Cancer
13. Stroke
14. Lupus

15. Hepatitis
16. Tuberculosis
17. Skin problems
18. Eye problems
19. Thyroid problems
20. Heart problems
21. Lung problems
22. Gall bladder problems
23. Kidney problems
24. Gastrointestinal problems
25. Blood or clotting problems
26. Liver problems
27. HIV disease
28. Organ transplant

29. Varicella

30. Chlamydia
31. Condyloma
32. Gonorrhea
33. Hepatitis B
34. Herpes
35. Syphilis
36. Pelvic inflammatory disease (PID)
37. Abnormal Pap smear
38. A vaginal infection (yeast, trichomonas, bacterial vaginosis [BV])
39. Abnormal vaginal bleeding
40. Pelvic pain
41. Urinary incontinence
42. Incontinence of feces or flatus
43. Infertility

44. Surgery (When/kind/reason/complications)
45. Accidents/injuries/trauma
46. Any blood products? When/kind/reason
47. Any hospitalizations? When/reason/complications

48. What medicines have you taken in the past?
49. Drug allergies? Other allergies?

50. Depression
51. Anxiety
52. Panic feelings
53. Mood swings
54. Nervous breakdown
55. Suicidal
56. Ever had counseling?

(continued)

> **Box 2-2. Data to be Obtained for the Medical/Surgical History** (Continued)
>
> **57.** Participated in a self-help group
> **58.** Ever been on medication for your nerves or a mental problem?
> **59.** Ever been hospitalized for a nervous or mental problem?
> **60.** An eating disorder or history of dieting
>
> **61.** Problems in regard to having or enjoying sex including pain, lack of desire, lack of orgasm
>
> **62.** History of sexual, physical, emotional abuse
>
> **63.** Visits to a naturopath, chiropractor, hypnotist, acupuncturist, herbalist, or traditional healer for health care or disease prevention?
> **64.** Use of vitamins, teas, tinctures, salves or ointments, acupuncture, biofeedback, chiropractic, energy healing, folk remedies, spiritual or religious healing, herbal or plant medicine, homeopathy, hypnosis, guided imagery, massage, or relaxation techniques, to treat or prevent illness?

Box 2-3 lists the criteria for Major Depressive Episode.

Eating Disorders

Women who have a history of an eating disorder may fear gaining weight while they are pregnant. This applies whether they are or have been diagnosed with anorexia nervosa, bulimia nervosa (either purging or non-purging), or binge-eating disorder (bingeing), a new diagnosis made when

> **Box 2-3. Criteria for Major Depressive Episode**
>
> For major depressive disorder, at least five of the following symptoms are present during the same time period, and at least one of the first two symptoms must be present. In addition, symptoms must be present most of the day, nearly daily, for at least 2 weeks.
>
> - Depressed mood most of the day, nearly every day
> - Markedly diminished interest or pleasure in almost all activities most of the day, nearly every day (as indicated either by subjective account or observation by others of apathy most of the time)
> - Significant weight loss/gain
> - Insomnia/hypersomnia
> - Psychomotor agitation/retardation
> - Fatigue (loss of energy)
> - Feelings of worthlessness (guilt)
> - Impaired concentration (indecisiveness)
> - Recurrent thoughts of death or suicide
>
> Source: American Psychiatric Association, 1987.

the criteria for bulimia nervosa are fulfilled but vomiting, laxatives, fasting or excessive exercise are not regularly used to compensate for binge eating. A binge is defined as eating an excessive amount of food within a 2-hour period and feeling unable to control what or how much is consumed. This must occur an average of twice a week for at least 3 months to be considered binge eating.

When you inquire about a history of eating disorders, you may find that this is a good time to talk about weight gain in pregnancy. You could begin by asking "What is your usual weight?" and follow with "Is this what you would like to weigh? What do you think is your ideal weight? How much do you think you would like to gain while you are pregnant?" The babies of pregnant women who have an eating disorder may not receive essential nutrients and women may suffer from both guilt over not feeding the baby properly and stress from feeling fat. Counseling can be helpful.

Foreign Travel or Residence

A travel and residential history may suggest the need for certain kinds of testing. For example, in certain countries parasites, malaria, hepatitis or tuberculosis are endemic. Women who have visited or lived in these areas should receive appropriate testing.

Sexual History

A sexual history is part of a complete data base because it may provide important medical information, give the clinician a more complete understanding of the client, and provide opportunities to (1) identify a client with a history of sexual abuse; (2) offer information that may relieve anxiety and dispel myths; (3) offer suggestions to improve sexual functioning; and (4) make referrals when sexual dysfunction or emotional problems are noted.

Asking Questions About Sex

While sexual problems are prevalent among both men and women who seek medical care, clinicians may have a difficult time initiating a discussion about sexual matters. A time-consuming interview that encompasses every aspect of a person's sexuality is not necessary for most situations encountered in the clinic or office. All that is necessary is basic information about sexuality and sexual problems, knowledge of one's own values regarding sexual behavior, a nonjudgmental attitude toward individuals with different values, and an attitude that conveys not only a willingness to discuss aspects of sexuality and sexual behavior, but also a belief that this information is important.

You might consider prefacing your questions with "We know that many men and women have problems and questions in regard to sex. Often we are able to help. Can I ask you a few questions?" (Box 2-4)

Sexual Problems

Common concerns about sex in women include frequency of intercourse, lack of sexual desire, dyspareunia, preorgasmia, anxiety about sexual orientation, post-traumatic stress from sexual abuse, and problems within a relationship (Ende, Rockwood, & Glasgow, 1984). If a problem exists, determine whether or not it is a long-standing or a recent problem. How much of a problem is it? Does the client's partner recognize the problem? Does the client know the cause? What has she done about the problem?

> ## Box 2-4. Questions to Ask About Sex*
>
> 1. Are you currently sexually active? With more than one partner?
> 2. Are you having any problems with how often you have sex? (Or, if client is partnered, you might ask) "Do you and your partner agree on how often you have sex?"
> 3. What about problems with whether you have sex or not?
> 4. Is there any pain with insertion, or penetration, or thrusting? Any pain after intercourse?
> 5. Any problems having an orgasm?
> 6. Does your partner have any sexual problems?
> 7. Would you say you are satisfied or unsatisfied with the sexual part of your life? (You might ask her to rate this part of her life on a scale of 1 to 10.)
> 8. How satisfied do you think your partner is?
> 9. Is there anything you would like to change?
> 10. Is there something you think your partner would like to change?
> 11. Has your partner said anything about having sex with you since you've become pregnant?
>
> ---
> *Adapt these questions to individual situations.

Sometimes a concern can be solved by providing information, by assuring the client that her concern is a common one, or by telling her that activities she may feel anxious about are considered "normal." For example, a pregnant woman might feel relieved to know that some men prefer not to have sexual intercourse after a certain point in pregnancy because they are afraid it will hurt the baby. A woman may also appreciate knowing that many women notice a change in their desire for sex when they are pregnant. Sexual problems, however, are often a result of problems within the relationship itself, and a referral for counseling may be more appropriate.

History of Sexual Abuse

The sexual history should inquire about past or present sexual abuse. Sometimes asking "How old were you when you had your first sexual experience?" is a useful question with which to start. Follow with "Was this with or without your permission?" This question puts you in a position to inquire further about sexual abuse. You might continue by asking if she has had sex subsequently without her consent. Has she been forced to participate in any sexual activity against her will? Affirmative responses to these questions can be emotionally intense for both the client and the clinician, particularly when the clinician has a personal history of childhood sexual abuse. (See Appendix H for some appropriate responses.)

Information about sexual abuse is important because memories of the abuse can surface during a pelvic examination as well as in labor or during breastfeeding. Share this information with clients who reveal a history of sexual abuse and ask the client if she would be willing to talk with you a bit more about it. Add that you would like to talk to her about what she might do if this happens. You might also tell her that major changes in a woman's life, such as pregnancy, may bring up issues from the past. Let her know that you are always ready to listen and can serve as a resource should questions or concerns surface. Respect the desires of the client who will not share her story with you at this time. It is inappropriate to destroy defense mechanisms, such as denial, that help a woman cope with her life.

History and Presence of Physical or Emotional Abuse

Questions about sexual abuse logically lead into questions about physical and emotional abuse. This information is considered important because abuse can start or get worse during pregnancy (Helton, McFarlane, & Anderson, 1987). "... there is reason to believe that violence may be a more common problem for pregnant women than preeclampsia, gestational diabetes, and placenta previa, conditions for which pregnant women are routinely screened and evaluated" (Gazmararian et al, 1996, p. 1920). Not only will there be psychological and bodily harm to the expectant mother in these cases, but trauma to the maternal abdomen may cause premature separation of the placenta and death of the baby. Study after study identifies routine screening of pregnant women for abuse as both appropriate and important.

> *Pregnancy is our window of opportunity to form a partnership with every woman to offer assessment, advocacy, and resources to prevent potential and existing abuse. Straightforward assessment readily identifies abuse during pregnancy. Not to assess for abuse is to deny the pregnant woman an opportunity to prevent additional abuse and possible trauma. Assessment for abuse during pregnancy must be standard of care for all pregnant women (McFarlane, 1992, p. 360).*

Asking questions about abuse in pregnancy may help women identify for the first time that they are, indeed, being abused. This may be particularly true for women "... immersed in cultures that grant men the implicit right to control and censure their behavior" (Olavarietta & Sotelo, 1996, p. 1937). Gender violence occurs throughout the life cycle. In addition to the physical, emotional, and sexual abuse common in the United States, gender violence includes sex-selective abortion, infanticide, genital mutilation, child marriage, acid throwing for purposes of revenge, bride burning when a dowry is considered inadequate, and wife burning upon the death of a husband in some countries.

It is often difficult for clinicians to appreciate the powerful emotional barriers that prevent women from leaving abusive relationships. Lack of financial support, a belief that children should be raised in a family with a father, and religious doctrine that speaks against separation or divorce are common. Other barriers are fear of the police, guilt, embarrassment, love for the offender, feeling that the abuse is deserved, and a belief that the offender will change. Perhaps most powerful is the realistic fear of retaliation.

Clinicians may find it particularly difficult to understand why some women refuse to go to a domestic violence shelter. Unfortunately, however, life in a shelter is not easy. The rules may be difficult to abide by, the environment is often chaotic, and some shelters will not house male children over the age of 10. Some shelters require a commitment to leaving the relationship. Pets are rarely permitted, leaving women fearful for their pets' safety should they leave.

Clinicians who work with women in abusive situations should not focus on the client leaving the situation when leaving is not the option that the client wishes to pursue. If she agrees to counseling, be sure that it is freely chosen. Avoid suggesting therapy and court mediation to couples because the immediate issue is *not* marital conflict and because court mediation operates on the assumption that two people are equal parties who can negotiate in good faith and arrive at a reasonably equitable solution. Such an assumption is erroneous when applied to an abuser and his victim and reflects ignorance of the dynamics of battering (Fish, 1989).

Clinicians should be informed about community resources for domestic violence, rape crisis, and abuse counseling. Both the National Coalition Against Domestic Violence and the National Coalition Against Sexual Assault are sources of information about local programs. (For their phone numbers, see Appendix F.)

Nontraditional Healing Practices

Many people look outside the traditional health care system for alleviation of their symptoms. As many as 1 in 4 Americans seeing a physician for a serious health problem may also be using nontraditional therapy (Eisenberg et al, 1993). Women who use these alternative and complementary practices represent all social classes and educational levels.

To have a more complete picture of the client's approach to health care and to identify potentially harmful practices, inquire about the client's use of nonmedical doctors and nontraditional therapies such as chiropractic, homeopathy, acupuncture and acupressure, massage, exercise, hypnosis, vitamin therapy, relaxation techniques and biofeedback, spiritual healing and prayer, lifestyle diets such as macrobiotics or vegan, imagery, herbs, weight-loss programs, self-help groups, energy healing, and folk remedies.

Medicines

Ask the client about use of past and present prescription and over-the-counter drugs. Inquire about drug allergies, including a description of any reaction that occurs following ingestion of the drug. Fortunately, only a few drugs are known to cause birth defects. (Box 2-5.) Box 2-6 lists the Food and Drug Administration's (FDA's) categorization of drugs in pregnancy.

Inquire specifically about vitamin supplements and nontraditional remedies. Ask clients to bring vitamin containers to the prenatal visit to document their content.

Family History

Information about the client's family is important to identify women at risk for having a genetic disease that could affect the outcome of pregnancy, or for having a child with a genetic disease. This information can also identify a racial or ethnic background needing an approach that takes into consideration a cultural heritage different from that of the health care provider or an increased risk for organic disease that may have a hereditary component.

The provider should also determine whether or not

- There is a family history of psychiatric illness (including depression) or alcohol or drug abuse

Box 2-5. Medications Associated with Adverse Fetal Effects

ACE inhibitor	Renal insufficiency oliguria
Acetylsalicylic acid	Intracranial hemorrhage, growth retardation
Alcohol	Microcephaly, growth retardation, short nose, hypoplastic maxilla, cardiac defects
Aminopterin methotrexate	Meningoencephalocele, hydrocephalus, brachy-cephaly, growth retardation
Carbamazepine	Meningomyelocele, cardiac defects, nasal hypoplasia
Warfarin	Nasal hypoplasia, skeletal deformities, congenital heart disease, stippled epiphysis, chondroplastia punctata, growth retardation, bleeding
Daunorubicin	Anencephaly, cardiac defects
Lithium	Cardiac defects
Methyl mercury	Microcephaly
Phenytoin	Congenital cardiac defects, microcephaly, hypoplastic distal phalanges, growth retardation
Propylthiouracil, methimazole	Goiter, cutis aplasia
Quinolones	Cartilagenous erosions
Retinoic acid	Congenital heart defects, hydrocephalus, micro-cephaly, limb deformities
Tetracycline	Limb deformities, yellow deciduous teeth
Trimethadione	Microcephaly, cardiac defects, club foot, growth re-tardation
Valproic acid	Meningomyelocele, microcephaly, tetralogy of Fallot, nasal hypoplasia, low-set ears

From Dacus, J.V., Meyer, N.L., & Sibai, B.M. (1995). How preconception counseling improves pregnancy outcome. *Contemporary OB/GYN, 40*(6), 115.

- The client's mother or a sister has had severe preeclampsia
- The client's mother took DES when the client was in utero.

Risk for Genetic Disease

Increased risk for genetic disease may be identified by inquiring about a family history of organic and psychiatric diseases that have a genetic component; ethnic background; and the presence of birth defects, mental retardation, infertility (as opposed to no children by choice), neonatal or infant deaths, and an unusual number of spontaneous abortions (see Box 1-1).

Ethnic Background

Race, ethnic and cultural heritage should be identified to provide clients with culturally sensitive care, and to identify women or families with autosomal recessive conditions with a high incidence in specific populations. If such conditions are identified, these women should be offered genetic screening.

Ask the client if anyone in her family or the family of the baby's father has a birth defect. Certain diseases and birth defects, as discussed previously, run in

Box 2-6. FDA Categories for Drugs in Pregnancy

Category A: No risk to fetus in first trimester demonstrated in controlled studies, and no evidence of risk in other trimesters.

Category B: No fetal risk shown in animal studies but no controlled studies in pregnant women are available, or animal studies showed an adverse effect *not* confirmed in controlled studies with pregnant women in the first trimester.

Category C: Adverse effects on fetus found in animal studies but no controlled studies in women, or studies in women and animals are not available. Give drug only if the benefit justifies the possible risk to the fetus.

Category D: Positive evidence of fetal risk exists but the benefits may be acceptable despite the risk, as in life-threatening situations or serious disease.

Category X: Fetal abnormalities have been demonstrated or evidence for fetal risk exists, and use of the drug outweighs any benefit.

Source: U.S. Food and Drug Administration

families. Obtain as much information as possible about the defect. Ask if there is anyone with mental retardation. When two or more family members are affected or dysmorphic features are present, a genetics consultation should be recommended.

Ask also about diseases that run in the family. A positive response is particularly important when two or more close relatives are affected. If anyone in the family has had a stillborn baby or has had a baby die early in life, realize that the stillbirth may be due to an unrecognized genetic disorder, and the neonatal death may indicate an inheritable metabolic disorder. The latter may have been erroneously attributed to SIDS, particularly if the death occurred before the age of 1 month or after the age of 12 months. Finish by asking "Is there any chance that you and your partner are blood-related?" Only consanguinity in the pregnant couple matters. If either member of the expectant couple is the product of a consanguineous relationship and is genetically normal, no increased risk for genetic disease exists.

Cultural Sensitivity

Cultural sensitivity begins in the heart of the health care provider who, hopefully, rejoices in the customs, perspectives, and approaches to living brought by women of different traditions. It includes recognizing that immigrant women, in particular, often come to the United States because of political repression, persecution and civil war, economic stagnation and extreme poverty, or religious repression and persecution. Those experiences suggest that these women may not only bring suffering and vulnerable spirits but also a lack of exposure to independent decision-making. Knowledge of the economic, religious, and sociopolitical aspects of ethnic communities, as well as the individual woman's story (if she is willing to share it), should be a high priority for clinicians fortunate enough to serve women and families of varied backgrounds. Also important is information about common methods of communication; beliefs about health, illness, and family structure; and beliefs about the role of the clinician, the client, and the family in decision-making.

Inadvertent assumptions about lifestyle, work habits, interpersonal relationships, values, activities of daily living, and convictions, particularly as the latter relate to health practices and beliefs about illness, can become barriers between cultures. Practitioners can be effective when they know the possibilities for discordance between their own health beliefs and those of women with different cultural backgrounds, and when they work to increase their knowledge about cultural beliefs, practices, and traditions that can affect a person's response to illness, the preferred treatment, and the health care provider.

Problems can also arise when the clinician needs to obtain "informed consent" from a woman of another culture. Imagine the dilemma posed in situations where the client is of a culture in which a person is identified primarily as a member of a family or community. The American concern for individual autonomy can run right into a cultural belief that family members should be the primary decision-makers about a client's treatment.

Imagine another scene in which the clinician provides a lengthy list of benefits, risks, side effects, and complications associated with a procedure. Truthtelling and full disclosure are the hallmarks of informed consent in the United States. But in other cultures it is believed that talking about adverse events can make them happen. We must approach these situations with caution and with recognition of our own cultural values.

Box 2-7 lists information that may help clinicians respond sensitively to clients of a different culture.

Clinicians should recognize that there is no generic Asian or Latino population, even though each may be grouped that way. *Hispanic,* a term used by the United States government for statistical purposes, may be less desirable to some people than *Latina,* partially because *Hispanic* connotes Spanish ancestry and ignores the African and indigenous heritage of people from Central and South America. *Latina* also ignores African and indigenous heritage, but is preferred by some over *Hispanic.* In fact, neither term is perfect and, for that reason, country of origin may be the best choice. It can also be helpful to follow country of origin with "American" when the person was born in the United States (eg, Mexican American).

When more than one term may be applied to a person's ethnic background, ask the client how she would like to be described: "Do you like to be described as Indian or as Native American?" "Do you like to be called Hispanic or Latina, black or African American?"

Interpreters

When clients speak another language, this barrier can have a profound effect on care. The usual clues of nonverbal communication familiar to clinicians—eye contact, affect, gestures and hand movements—may be absent, and unintended meanings may unintentionally offend. Even clinicians who have learned the language of non–English-speaking clients have problems when they have not been raised in the client's culture. Nuances may be missed, appropriate ways of phrasing sensitive questions may be unknown, and important aspects of the culture may remain hidden.

Some problems arising from a language barrier can be minimized when a translator or interpreter is available. In ideal situations this person is bicultural as well as bilingual, is familiar with medical terminology, and has had special training in cross-cultural interpretation.

Box 2-7. Information that Can Help Clinicians Respond Sensitively to Clients of a Different Culture

1. What is the appropriate form of address? (First names may not be appropriate.)
2. What greetings are appropriate? Should the greeting be different according to status? Should the greeting be lengthy? Include social chit chat?
3. Are there any restrictions on the sex of the person providing care?
4. Are there any customs to be observed in regard to eye contact?
5. To what extent should the partner, extended family, or the community be involved in decision-making?
6. Are there any restrictions on who may touch whom? On body parts that should not be touched? On body contact between the sexes?
7. Are pelvic examinations likely to cause particular embarrassment? What can be done to lessen this embarrassment?
8. Should any special practices be observed during pregnancy? Labor? Birth? Any rituals? Special clothes, amulets to wear? Certain foods to eat or not eat? Taboos to observe?
9. Should special medicines, herbs, teas, poultices, or treatments be used?
10. Are any other practitioners consulted during pregnancy or after delivery? Who are they? What do they do?
11. Does pregnancy change usual sexual practices? Hygiene practices? Patterns of work?
12. What persons or practices are considered dangerous to either the pregnant woman or her baby? What is done about them?
13. What special practices should be observed after delivery? Special food? Special place for the mother?

---

* Adapted from Office of International Health, U.S. Public Health Service. *Guidelines for analysis of sociocultural factors in health.* (1989).

The interpreter should also be of similiar educational and social class. If the client is from a lower class, he or she may be intimidated, and if the client is from a higher class, the client may doubt the abilities of the interpreter or may refrain from full disclosure of health care issues (Poss & Rangel, 1995, p. 44).

Use of an interpreter from the same country as the client is also helpful.

All people who speak the same language do not necessarily communicate well. For example, Spanish speakers from different countries or of different educational backgrounds will not necessarily understand each other. An interpreter who speaks Spanish as it is spoken in Spain will not communicate well with a person from rural Mexico. There are countless stories about misunderstandings between Spanish speakers from different countries. For instance, guagua means "bus" in Puerto Rico, but it means "baby" in Chile. Misunderstandings can occur with the word biscocho, which means "cake" to someone from Puerto Rico but is slang for female genitals to a Mexican (Poss & Rangel, 1995, p. 44).

While it is impossible to have a fully qualified interpreter always available, clinicians should be aware of the limitations of a given situation. A particularly difficult encounter will involve choices with which the interpreter cannot morally agree, or a subject that makes the encounter uncomfortable. In these situations, the interpreter may interject personal values.

For example, a clinician wanted to ask a client if she wanted to use a method of birth control. After the clinician posed the question, the interpreter responded "No, she doesn't," without asking the client. Another clinician, wanting to ask a woman if she was in an abusive situation, spoke enough Spanish to understand that the interpreter said "Your husband doesn't hit you, does he?" (See Appendix I for guidelines for working with an interpreter.)

At times it is necessary to ask a family member to serve as an interpreter. When this occurs, be aware of the potentially embarrassing situation for both the interpreter and the client. Be aware, as well, that the information obtained may be superficial or inaccurate.

Risk for Organic or Psychiatric Disease

Organic diseases with a hereditary component include some forms of heart disease (heart attacks before age 55 in men and before age 65 in women), diabetes, certain breast cancers, and colon cancer. While these conditions are rare occurrences in pregnant women, they can occur. Information about their presence in a family should be recorded for discussion at a later time. The postpartum visit is often an appropriate time to discuss preventive measures and plan for follow-up. Certain psychiatric disorders are also known to have a hereditary component.

Abuse in the Family

Recently, researchers in the field of abuse have pointed out that a child who observes a family member being abused automatically experiences emotional abuse. Asking about violence in the family and whether or not any family member observed such occurrences as part of the family history can provide an opportunity to begin asking questions about the client's personal experience with all forms of violence.

Abuse of Alcohol and Illicit Drugs

Ask about the use of alcohol and drugs by close family members of the client. Sometimes inquiring "Has alcohol (or drugs) affected your life in any way?" opens the door to a fruitful discussion of this topic.

Adoption

If the client was adopted, this may be a good time to ask how that experience has affected her. For some people, adoption has been wonderful. For others it has always been painful. Pregnancy is often the factor that motivates a man or a woman to wonder about family background. Ask the client who has been adopted (and, when possible, the baby's father, if the father has been adopted) if she has thought of "searching" for her birth parents. People who decide to try to find their birth parents need to know that much joy and much pain can come from reuniting. Often, help from a counselor who has experience in the field of adoption can be helpful in making a decision about whether or not to "search."

Environmental Exposures

Toxic Agents

Most people are unaware of the degree of their exposure to harmful agents. Exposure is usually due to one's place of residence or occupation. In some cases, a test to measure the blood level of certain elements, such as lead and mercury, is indicated. (Appendix C contains sample exposure questions.)

X-rays During the Current Pregnancy

Any exposure to radiation may carry the risk of genetic effects and birth defects. However, exposures that involve less than 5 rads are not associated with congenital malformations. Most diagnostic studies involve a low radiation exposure. Computer tomography (CT) scans give the most radiation. (An abdominal CT series equals 2.6 rads, while a chest x-ray equals .008 rads). However, a CT is sometimes necessary to evaluate a client for trauma subsequent to an injury.

Significant exposures to x-rays in utero may increase the risk for childhood cancer. Research suggests that ". . . the most sensitive period of exposure for developing leukemia is about the seventh month of pregnancy. The most sensitive period of exposure for developing all cancers, except leukemia, is the first six months of pregnancy" (Hanford Health Information Network, 1994, p. 5).

Habits Undermining Health

Smoking

Most women know that they should not smoke when they are pregnant, though they may not know exactly what the hazards are. Women who smoked in previous pregnancies and gave birth to healthy babies may not believe there really are risks. Some women, thinking their labor will be easier or shorter, like the idea of having a smaller baby. Some like the way smoking helps them decrease anxiety, relieve tension, or keep their weight down.

Because many women are willing to make sacrifices for their children and many women would like to quit smoking, pregnancy is an excellent time to ask women to stop. Advice from a health care provider combined with support and self-help materials can be a powerful motivator.

While some practitioners feel that stopping smoking is something that is under the expectant mother's control and a responsibility that she has toward her unborn child, smoking cessation is not easy and not always something that a woman can freely choose to do. Knowledge and motivation are not all that is needed for a woman to stop. Studies have shown that continuing to smoke may be a mother's way of reconciling the needs of the unborn baby with the needs of the family as a whole. Smoking may provide a harried mother with a few minutes each day to herself and the ability to stay calm; it may be the only thing that she does for herself all day. Women who are substance abusers may use smoking to help them from using other drugs. ". . . Noncompliance with medical advice may reflect not so much a failing on the part of the mother as her superior knowledge of the constraints of everyday family life" (Graham, 1988). See Box 2-8 for questions that can be helpful in understanding a woman's smoking habit.

Once you know that a client smokes, ask "What do you know about smoking in pregnancy?" Many women do not know exactly what effects

Box 2-8. Questions to Ask About Smoking

1. How many people that you live with smoke?
2. Does _____ (name of person closest to her) smoke too?
3. What brand do you smoke?
4. How many cigarettes do you smoke a day?
5. Do you smoke marijuana also? (Ask how much if the answer is yes.)
6. How soon after waking do you have your first cigarette?
7. Have you ever tried to stop before? If yes, what happened?
8. How old were you when you started smoking?
9. Do you know why you smoke?
10. How is smoking affecting you?

smoking can have on the baby. Use of a prenatal smoking cessation protocol such as the one developed by the Colorado Department of Public Health and Environment, *Smoking cessation in pregnancy: Counseling protocols for doctors and nurses,* can be useful. The Colorado project shows how to take just 1 to 3 minutes at each prenatal visit to assess the client's smoking habit and, for those wishing to quit, evaluate progress toward that goal. Copies of the protocol can be obtained by writing to Nancy Salas, Colorado Department of Public Health and Environment, PPD-ASSIS-A5, 4300 Cherry Creek South, Denver, CO 80222-1530. The department also makes available camera-ready art for several two-sided handouts they have designed (in conjunction with the Centers for Disease Control and Prevention) for women who are trying to stop smoking. The handouts are entitled *Give a gift to your baby, Keep your baby smoke free,* and *To slip and smoke doesn't mean you've failed.* The art can be borrowed for 30 days, allowing time to have the sheets printed and personalized. (Write to Deb Fowler at the above address, or phone 303/692-2516.)

The National Cancer Institute publishes *How to help your patients stop smoking: A National Cancer Institute manual for physicians.* For a free copy (one per caller), call 1-800-4-CANCER.

Alcohol

The significant problems posed by children with fetal alcohol syndrome and alcohol-related neurodevelopmental disorder make it imperative that clinicians ask about alcohol intake and remind women of the potential lifelong effect alcohol may have on the unborn baby (see Box 1-3 for suggested questions).

Since pregnant women, particularly heavy drinkers, often underreport alcohol intake, you might simply ask the client "How much do you drink?" To any response other than "Never," ask "How much do you drink in a week?" Suggest a few amounts, and start high, "A case, a few 6-packs?" If it is obvious that the client drinks on a daily basis, try "How much do you drink in a day—two packs? One?" Since alcoholism often leads to problems in many areas of the alcoholic's life, try to determine whether or not effects have been noticed in physical health, emotional well-being, relationships, the legal arena, and on the job or at school.

Illicit and Recreational Drugs

Identifying drug use in pregnancy is important for at least three reasons: to get help for women who wish to stop using; to identify fetuses and babies at risk; and to identify women at risk for human immunodeficiency virus (HIV) infection. Women using drugs cannot get help unless they are identified. If the clinician fails to ask about drug use, the perception on the part of the provider is likely to be a phenomenon known as NIMO (not in my office). These clinicians believe their clients do not use drugs.

It is true that it is often difficult to deal with responses when a woman is asked about drug use. Women who use drugs put a high priority on keeping their world safe. They keep secrets, minimize the extent of their use, and may take an aggressive stance, particularly when they view the health care provider as an obstacle. But a conspiracy of secrecy—you don't ask me, I won't tell you—serves no one. See Box 1-3 for suggested questions about drug use.

If the new mother continues using drugs after her baby is born, risk to the baby continues. Not only are the babies born biologically vulnerable, but they also are born to mothers who face health and emotional problems of their own. These women are compromised in their ability to establish relationships and may be unable to respond to the baby's needs, particularly if they receive an infant who is medically fragile after an extensive hospital stay.

Many women who are chemically addicted experience intense guilt about their drug use and live in fear that their baby will be taken from them. Identifying drug- and alcohol-using pregnant women can change a woman's life. It can mean a full life for mother and baby instead of one in which the baby experiences developmental delay, retardation, or even death. Not all women, of course, will be able to change a lifestyle that involves the use of drugs because they are pregnant. However, a woman may be able to choose a different path later, because of a seed you planted.

Social History

Family Constellation

Information about the client's family should include her family of origin, place of birth, the people with whom she is living, the people that she considers "family," and the people that she can count on for support. You might ask "Could you tell me a little bit about the important people in your life?" or "Whom do you include in your immediate family?" The client's response can lead to questions about a partner, parents, siblings, other relatives, and friends.

You might continue with "Do you live with a partner?" or "Are you single, partnered, married, separated, divorced, or widowed?," indicating that you are aware that not all pregnant women are involved in a conventional marriage arrangement. Ask about the quality of relationships with the partner or with the father of the baby if the baby's father is not the client's partner. The 1-to-10 scale can be helpful for some women: "On a scale of 1-to-10, with 10 being a wonderful relationship and 1 being an awful relationship, where would you put your relationship now?" Unless the answer is "10," follow with "What would it take to make it a 10?" You might also ask, "Can you count on your partner to be there for you?" Inquire about relationships with parents, siblings, friends, and with the partner's family as well.

If a woman who is a lesbian informs you about her sexual orientation, ask whether or not her sexual preference is known to family, friends and coworkers, and whether or not she wants information about her sexuality in her medical record. Lesbians vary greatly in where they are in the "coming out" process and in their need for confidentiality. Nonjudgmental, sensitive health care by providers who are knowledgeable about lesbians, aware of their anxiety and vulnerability in traditional heath care settings, and willing to discuss their needs in regard to secrecy, support, and referrals will be appreciated.

Living Situation

Obtain information about where the client lives, how often she has moved, the kind of dwelling she lives in, the number of people, the safety of the area, and when indicated, whether or not there is sufficient food in the house.

Occupation

Knowing the client's occupation is important in order to know the client in a holistic way as well as to assess the potential for preterm birth and for exposure to occupational hazards that might damage the fetus. Data to support recommendations about limiting or eliminating certain kinds of work experience for women are not available. However, women whose jobs require standing or walking for more than 5 hours per day may have an increased rate of preterm birth (Henriksen et al, 1995). Exposure to high noise levels and some forms of shift work may also increase the incidence of preterm birth as well as low birth weight and spontaneous abortion (Nurminen, 1995).

Job requirements may expose employees to metals, dust, fibers, fumes, chemicals, biologic hazards, noise, vibration, and radiation. Ask about health practices used on the job site. Be aware of associations between job category and exposure to agents such as insecticides, herbicides, and fungicides used in agriculture. Unfortunately, most attempts to study the influences of occupation and environment on reproduction do not control for exposure to multiple factors that could account for study findings. Nevertheless, it is important to consider the dangers potentially posed by occupation and fluctuating work hours.

Occupation is also important, as it provides some information about income level. Data from the 1988 National Maternal and Infant Health Survey (the most recent data available) found that the infant mortality rate was 60% higher, and the postneonatal mortality rate twice as high, for women living below the poverty level than for women whose incomes were above the poverty level. (See Box 2-9 for the Federal Poverty Guidelines.) Most of the postneonatal deaths

Box 2-9. Federal Poverty Guidelines: April 1, 1995–June 30, 1996			
Family Size	100% FPL Monthly	133% FPL Monthly	185% FPL Monthly
1	$ 623	$ 828	$1152
2	836	1112	1547
3	1049	1395	1941
4	1263	1679	2336
5	1476	1963	2731
6	1689	2247	3125
7	1903	2530	3520
8	2116	2814	3915

were for infectious diseases or injuries. Low income level should be added to adolescent pregnancy, smoking, late entry into or poor utilization of prenatal care, low educational level, and nondominant race or ethnic group as a social or behavioral characteristic that increases a woman's risk for poor perinatal outcome (CDC, 1995c). (See Box 2-10 for suggested questions about occupation.)

The client's responses to inquiries about occupation can help the provider be aware of services and benefits that might be available to the client and her family. The Women, Infants, and Children (WIC) program, for example, is a health and nutrition program for pregnant women, breastfeeding women, and young children. The program provides health and nutrition information, supplemental food, and access to health care services for pregnant women, nursing mothers (for up to 12 months after delivery), and children from birth to age 5. Pregnant women receive milk, cheese, eggs, vitamin C-fortified fruit juices, iron-fortified cereal, and peanut butter, dried beans or peas, or lentils. Breastfeeding mothers also receive carrots, canned tuna, peanut butter *and* peas, beans, or lentils for themselves. Women who are not breastfeeding receive infant formula for the first 12 months of the baby's life. Eligibility is based on a household income that is 185% or less of the federal poverty level.

Education, Interests, Hobbies, and Goals

Ask about the highest grade that the client has completed, as well as her interests, hobbies, and long-term goals. This information helps the clinician understand the client as a person and provides some insight into her literacy level. Occasionally, potential hazards from hobbies such as painting, sculpting, welding, woodworking, piloting, auto racing, firearms, stained glass, ceramics, and gardening will be identified. Materials used in arts and crafts can contain silicon, talc, solvents, and heavy metals, all of which are potentially dangerous.

Religious Preference

Inquire about religious preference and any practices related to religion that should be observed. This information can lead to a discussion about the importance of religion in the client's life, religious traditions surrounding pregnancy

---

Box 2-10. Questions to Ask About Occupation

1. Are you working now for money? Tell me a little about the job—what you do, the hours you work, how many days a week.
2. How much standing does your job involve?
3. Have you ever worked with or around anything that might be a health hazard? Ever had a job where you wore protective clothing?
4. Is there anything about your job that you think might be dangerous to you or your baby?
5. How do you like your job? Could you rate it on a scale of 1 to 10, with 1 being awful and 10 being terrific?
6. Do you make more than _____ each month? (See Box 2-9 and insert the figure that defines 100% of poverty based on the size of this woman's family.)

and birth, and feelings about the sex of the health care provider, and in some cases, the use of blood products.

Pets

Ask about the kind and number of pets in the dwelling. The potential for harm from dangerous pets, and the potential for illness from large numbers of pets, should be discussed.

Sources of Support

Inquire about the people the client can depend on for support. At times women will report that no one is available to them. More frequent and longer visits that focus on providing emotional support and establishing linkages with appropriate community resources should be scheduled, if possible.

Sources of Stress

Common sources of stress for pregnant women include money, housing, a difficult child, and relationship problems with a partner or other family member. Asking "What are your major sources of stress right now?" helps the clinician understand some of the factors impinging on the client's life.

Each clinician should develop a list of questions suitable for obtaining the information needed for the social history. Some questions are essential to ask. Others are not *essential* but help you understand the factors that affect the client's life and her ability to parent. For example, asking the client about her living situation allows you to determine whether or not her need for shelter is met and whether or not she feels safe. If the client is homeless or in a temporary residence, flagging the chart can help you remember to search for resources in the community that might be helpful, as well as to verify address and contact number at every visit.

Box 2-11 lists questions that can serve as a starting point for obtaining the social history. Adapt them to your personal style.

Health Promoting Habits

Information about the client's health habits will identify areas in which health education may be appropriate now or postpartally.

Safety

Inquire about the client's regular use of seat belts and protective gear and whether she engages in sports such as cycling, rollerblading, and riding all-terrain vehicles. Ask about the presence of smoke alarms and the last time that the batteries were changed. Remind women that a good time to change batteries is when they change the time on clocks at home, at the beginning and end of Daylight Savings Time.

Weapons of all kinds can be found in many homes and are increasingly carried by individuals. A 1990 study found that almost 20% of 9th through 12th-grade students had carried a weapon at least once in the preceding 30 days. Approximately 1 out of 20 students carried a handgun (CDC, 1991). Inquiring about the presence and method of storage of firearms in the home should be a

> **Box 2-11. Questions to Ask to Establish a Psychosocial Data Base**
>
> 1. Can you tell me a little about your childhood? Would you say that it was easy or hard?
> 2. Would you tell me a little about your mother? Your father? (step-parent, grandparent, as appropriate)
> 3. Did you have a nickname?
> 4. Was anyone in your house ever hit or put-down verbally?
> 5. Did you ever live with someone other than your mother or your father? If yes, what was that like?
> 6. Have you had any big losses in your life—a family member, a relationship, a job, moving?
> 7. How are you doing emotionally now?
> 8. How would you rate your life now on a scale of 1 to 10, with 1 being awful and 10 being terrific? What do you wish were different about your life?
>
> If not asked previously:
> 9. Have you ever had counseling? For how long (if yes)? For what reasons? Was it helpful? Why did you stop? Have you thought about getting more counseling?
> 10. Do you think you are depressed now?
>
> If adopted:
> 11. What has it been like, being adopted? Do you think about your birth parents? About "searching"?

routine part of a history. Anyone who is depressed, or who uses or lives with people using illicit drugs, should be advised to remove weapons for the protection of everyone.

Exercise

During pregnancy the influence of estrogen, progesterone, and elastin results in connective tissue laxity and joint instability. Some separation of the pubic symphysis is common. Nerve compression syndrome, as is found in carpal tunnel syndrome, may occur. These effects increase the likelihood of falling with resulting maternal injury and the possibility of premature separation of the placenta and preterm labor (PTL) if abdominal trauma occurs.

Concerns about exercise during pregnancy involve both mother and baby. These concerns include the potential for injury to both mother and fetus should a fall occur, and the consequences of an exercise program to the fetus. Women who do not engage in a regular exercise program may wonder if they should start one. Women already engaged in an exercise program may wonder about continuing. While specific health benefits (ie, shorter labors and fewer operative deliveries) from an exercise routine during pregnancy have not been documented by research studies, the psychological benefits some women experience as a result of an exercise program make it important to address the issues.

Concerns about fetal well-being relate to the theoretical potential for

- Fetal teratogenicity from fetal hyperthermia
- Hypoxia and intrauterine growth restriction from blood being shunted away from the maternal viscera to working muscles
- Preterm delivery.

In general, most clinicians feel that mild to moderate exercise during pregnancy is not harmful. Certain sports, however, seem to be inherently hazardous to pregnant women. A fall during water skiing could result in trauma to the abdomen or water under high pressure being forced into the vagina. Any contact sport could involve a fall or a blow to the abdomen. Orthopedic injuries from reduced joint stability and changes in equilibrium could also occur. Horseback riding, windsurfing, and diving also seem to pose undue risks because of their potential for trauma to the maternal abdomen. It seems prudent to advise women who run to avoid running when the temperature or humidity is unusually high.

Breast and Skin Examinations

Self breast examination is a practice that all women should be encouraged to perform monthly. Women between the ages of 35 and 40 should have a baseline mammogram, although this examination is not recommended during pregnancy unless a suspicious mass is noted, as the increased blood supply to the breasts during pregnancy makes mammograms difficult to interpret.

A skin check at the same time the breast examination is performed is an important health activity. Because of the association between solar rays and skin cancer, clients should be asked if they take any protective measures when they are in the sun. Use of tanning booths, another source of skin cancer, should be discouraged.

Immunizations

Asking pregnant women about previous immunizations is important to determine their need for initial vaccination or booster doses of certain vaccines post-partally.

Pregnant women who have not had chickenpox should be advised to stay away from anyone with this disease. They may wish to have a varicella titre-IgG drawn at the initial prenatal visit. If the IgG is positive, the client has had varicella. Women with a negative IgG who are exposed to varicella, should have a second titre drawn. If the IgG is still negative, varicella-zoster immunoglobulin (VZIG) should be administered within 96 hours of exposure. A pregnant woman who has never had chickenpox, has not had a varicella titre drawn, and is exposed to varicella should notify the health care provider immediately so that an initial varicella titre-IgG can be obtained.

It is common in certain developing countries to administer tetanus-diphtheria toxoid (Td) in the last trimester of pregnancy to protect babies against neonatal tetanus, the cause of an estimated 490,000 neonatal deaths in 1994 (CDC, 1996). While Td is considered safe in the second and third trimesters (Gall, 1995), it is not commonly offered to pregnant women in the United States because neonatal tetanus is practically nonexistent.

Hepatitis B vaccine is also considered safe in pregnancy. However, because pregnancy is a hypoimmune state with potential for infection of the fetus, some clinicians in developed countries prefer to administer vaccines after the baby is born. An exception to this is flu vaccine. Consideration should be given to offering influenza vaccine to women who will be in the third trimester of pregnancy or the puerperium during flu season (November to March) and pregnant women of any gestation who are at risk for influenza complications (CDC, 1995b). A 25% reduction in upper respiratory infections (URI), a 43% reduction in URI-related absenteeism from work, and a 44% reduction in office visits has been noted when nonpregnant, healthy adults were vaccinated against influenza (Nichol et al, 1995). There is no evidence of fetal risk at any gestational period with this vaccine. Protective titres are achieved about 2 weeks after vaccination and decline after 4 to 6 months. This vaccine should not be given to women who are allergic to eggs.

Health care providers should document all immunizations that clients have received so that appropriate recommendations can be made in the postpartum period. Certainly, health care providers should follow immunization recommendations for themselves as well as for their clients. While health care workers often think primarily of HIV infection when they observe universal precautions, hepatitis B infection is about 40 times more likely than HIV infection to occur after a needle stick (Zuckerman, 1995).

Nutrition

Common practice involves telling pregnant women what they *should* eat. It is less common to ask a woman what she *is* eating and what modifications, if any, she would like to initiate because of her pregnancy.

Dietary patterns are very hard to change. Perhaps most important during pregnancy is identifying women who will not or cannot consume enough calories to support good fetal growth. Women who fall into this category include women with pathologic morning sickness (hyperemesis gravidarum), women who are too poor to be able to buy enough food, women with an eating disorder, and women who have a problem with body image.

A discussion of nutrition can be initiated by asking "Is eating going to be an issue for you while you are pregnant?" This approach helps the clinician address what might be a concern for any woman. (See Box 2-12 for additional questions.) Be sure to inquire about nutritional supplements, particularly vitamins that are being consumed in lieu of or in addition to prenatal vitamins, if this subject has not been discussed previously. The potential for teratogenicity or for suppression of trace elements with high-dose vitamins should be considered.

If another person has remained with the client while you obtained the history, be sure to find some time to speak with the client alone. You might say to the person accompanying her "I'd like to speak with _____ alone for just a minute." At this time ask the client if there is anything else you should know about her in order to give her good care, anything confidential she wishes to tell you, or anything she has a question about.

Appendix K lists the topics appropriate to address when obtaining the initial visit history. You might want to copy the list onto a small card that you can place in front of you during the initial interview. Use the card to supplement the form used in your practice setting. After a few interviews, revise your card to reflect your own style and priorities.

Taking a good history takes a long time. The realities of the clinic and office situation do not permit enough time to ask all of the questions necessary to obtain the data desired. A form for the client to complete at home before the initial

> ### Box 2-12. Questions to Ask to Facilitate a Discussion
> ### of Weight Gain in Pregnancy
>
> **1.** What is your usual weight? Desired weight?
> **2.** Have you had a recent change in weight?
> **3.** Have you ever dieted? How often? What kind of diet? Most recent?
> **4.** Have you ever had an eating disorder—anorexia, bulimia?
> **5.** Number of meals per day
> **6.** Fluid intake per day, especially coffee, soda and milk
> **7.** Snack foods
> **8.** Foods not eaten and reason
> **9.** History of fasting? When? How long?
> **10.** Vitamin use: Kind, frequency, reason for taking
> **11.** If underweight, has this always been the case? Do you know why?
> **12.** If overweight, when did the weight problem begin? Does it run in the family? How much of a problem is it?
> **13.** Is eating going to be an issue for you while you are pregnant?
> **14.** How much weight do you think you should gain during this pregnancy?
> **15.** How much weight would you like to gain?

visit or at the clinic or office before being interviewed by the clinician can facilitate the history-taking procedure. Appendix L contains sample questions that may serve as a starting point for designing a form suitable to your approach and your practice setting. Women with low literacy skills may be unable to read or understand forms for clients to fill out, and women who speak no English will not be able to respond to forms written in English. In these instances, limit the questions asked at the first visit, saving some for subsequent visits.

Be sure to listen to other clinicians obtain client histories whenever you can. Each will emphasize different questions. Each will have a distinctive style. Listen to the way questions are phrased, how sensitive information is addressed, and the extent to which nonverbal cues are noted and used.

▼ The Physical Examination

The physical examination at the initial prenatal visit is intended to identify abnormalities most likely to contribute to morbidity and mortality, and to identify body features that suggest a genetic disorder. The examination should include determination of height and weight; measurement of blood pressure (BP) and pulse; an examination of the skin, thyroid gland, heart, lungs, breasts, extremities, and abdomen; and a pelvic examination. A chaperone should be present whenever possible to protect the interests of both client and provider. The chaperone's presence protects the client from inappropriate sexual advances, and the clinician from false charges of sexual impropriety. While most sexual impropriety occurs between male providers and female clients, same-sex boundary violations do occur.

Height

Short stature may be an indicator of a genetic disorder. Because exact height is often unknown and changes as women get older, height should be measured at the initial visit. When the client is shorter than expected for her family or when her height is more than two standard deviations below the mean, consult with a genetic counselor about the need for an evaluation for Turner's syndrome. A useful book for evaluating height in women living in developed countries who are of European descent is *Handbook of normal physical measurements* (Hall, J.B. et al, 1990, New York: Oxford University Press.)

Weight

Weight is obtained at the initial visit to recommend weight gain for the pregnancy and to track weight gain or loss. Over the years many suggestions have been made about the ideal weight gain for pregnant women. One source for current guidelines, the Institute of Medicine, uses Body Mass Index (BMI) to determine weight gain recommendations. The BMI is obtained by relating the client's height to her prepregnancy weight (Appendix M.) The Institute of Medicine recommends the following weight gains:

> 25 to 35 lb for women with a normal prepregnancy weight-for-height (BMI 19.8 to 26)
> 28 to 40 lb for underweight women (BMI less than 19.8)
> 15 to 25 lb for overweight women (BMI 26.1 to 29)
> at least 15 lb for obese women (BMI greater than 29)

(National Academy of Sciences, 1992).

Note that the weight gain goal is a range of pounds and uses the client's prepregnant weight as the basis for measuring gain, even though the weight reported by the client may not be accurate.

▶ SOMETHING FUN

> It can be fun for some women to weigh themselves and record the weight on a graph at each visit. Women with low literacy skills may find this activity difficult, and women who are obese or who have body-image problems may prefer not to participate.

Blood Pressure

Blood pressure (BP) determinations are important during pregnancy because elevations can endanger the lives of both mother and baby. In normal pregnancy, BP declines slightly as early as the 8th week. It stays down through the second trimester and then starts back toward prepregnant levels.

Measurement of blood pressure in pregnant women should follow standard techniques. Use an appropriately sized cuff, a properly calibrated manometer, an intact inflating system, and a stethoscope with tubing of an appropriate length. Remember that hearing acuity, visual acuity, concentration, the angle at which the meniscus of the mercury column is observed, the rate of inflation and deflation of the cuff, digit preference, and placement of the manometer will influence the accuracy of the reading.

A large measuring cuff usually should be used whenever the client's arm measures more than 35 cm around. If no large cuff is available, a regular cuff can be placed on the forearm. In this case the stethoscope should be placed over the radial artery. A small cuff used to determine blood pressure on a woman with a large arm is likely to give an erroneously high reading.

All BPs in pregnant women should be obtained with the woman in a sitting position. The same arm should be used each time, preferably the right arm for consistency. It is no longer accepted practice to have a woman with an elevated BP rest on her left side during the measurement. Blood pressures obtained this way give a low reading that can lead to false reassurance that the BP is within normal limits. Women with an elevated or slightly elevated BP in the first half of pregnancy may have chronic hypertension or, if nulliparous with a systolic reading of 120 mm Hg or greater, may be at risk for preeclampsia (Sibai, 1996).

In many prenatal settings the BP is obtained by someone other than the clinician. Because other BPs may be compared to early pregnancy measurements, it is a good idea to personally measure early pregnancy BPs.

Pulse

The maternal pulse increases slightly during pregnancy, but it is rarely over 100 beats per minute (bpm). Think of hyperthyroidism when it is over 100 bpm. Look for accompanying exophthalmos and hyperreflexia. When the pulse is over 100 bpm, order a free T3 or T4. Hyperthyroidism is not likely if tachycardia is absent.

Examination of the Skin

Common skin changes in pregnancy include hyperpigmentation of the face (chloasma), areola and nipples, striae gravidarum, spider nevi, and the linea negra. Examine the skin for color, rashes, growths, lesions, scars, signs of physical abuse, and evidence of intravenous drug use. Pay particular attention to a rash on the palms of the hands and soles of the feet that might be a sign of syphilis. Scars may be indicative of a surgical procedure or, in rare instances, to sexual practices associated with sadomasochistic rituals. When tattoos or piercings are present, ask about the needles used in the procedure. Shared needles can be a source of HIV infection. Six or more cafe-au-lait spots (CLS) equal to or greater than 15 mm in diameter may indicate neurofibromatosis.

Examination of the Thyroid Gland

The thyroid gland is slightly enlarged during pregnancy because of glandular hyperplasia and increased vascularity. These anatomic changes, however, do not produce significant thyromegaly, and any significant enlargement requires investigation. Hypothyroidism can be hard to detect in pregnancy because many of the symptoms of hypothyroidism—fatigue, weight gain, and constipation—mimic pregnancy.

Examination of the Lungs

The lung examination should include observing for shortness of breath, shallow breathing, rapid breathing, irregular respirations, guarded respirations, wheezing, coughing, and dyspnea. Healthy women rarely have lung problems. Examination of the lungs is usually most helpful to aid in a diagnosis of bronchitis or pneumonia. Listen for crackles, wheezes, and decreased breath sounds.

Examination of the Heart

Systolic heart murmurs may be found in as many as 90% of pregnant women (Cutforth & MacDonald, 1966). These murmurs result from the marked increase in blood volume that occurs in pregnancy—as much as 45% above a woman's nonpregnant level at the end of pregnancy (Pritchard, 1965). This increase nourishes the enlarged uterus and protects the mother when blood is lost at the time of birth.

In nonpregnant women, a systolic heart murmur may be significant. In an asymptomatic pregnant woman, a grade 1/6 or a grade 2/6 murmur is usually considered benign. When the systolic murmur is greater than 2/6, or if any other murmur is heard, request an echocardiogram if funds are available to perform this test. If funds are not available, request an electrocardiogram, and refer the client to a physician, if possible, for further evaluation.

Examination of the Breasts

The breasts should be examined for any breast mass that might be malignant and for conditions that could jeopardize breastfeeding. Be sure to examine the nipples carefully, especially if the client wishes to breastfeed. A test for "protractility" should be part of the prenatal breast examination for women who have not successfully breast-fed previously. With your thumb and forefinger, compress the breast tissue about one inch behind the areola. If the nipple projects forward, the baby will probably have no difficulty latching on.

Inverted and Flat Nipples

"Breast shells" to stretch inverted nipples may start at the 28th week. If the client has symptoms of PTL or has previously given birth to a preterm baby, delay breast shell use until 36 weeks' gestation because breast stimulation may provoke uterine contractions.

Flat nipples almost always occur in women with large breasts and are due to the weight of the breasts. Breast shells for flat nipples do not need to be used prenatally. Instead, instruct the mother to use them after delivery. Applying them to the nipples for about 20 minutes before infant feeding usually causes protrusion of the nipple for a short period of time. The baby should be put to breast as soon as they are removed.

Mammary Agenesis

One situation that precludes breastfeeding is mammary agenesis, the absence of breast tissue. On initial examination a woman with mammary agenesis may be thought to be merely "flat-chested." Close inspection and palpation will establish a diagnosis. Women with mammary agenesis will produce colostrum and, perhaps, a small amount of breast milk, but the amount will not be sufficient to nourish the baby.

Breast Reduction and Augmentation

Women who have had breast reduction or breast augmentation surgery may have problems with breastfeeding. Older surgical procedures for breast reduction involved reimplanting the nipple to make it look anatomically correct. Unfortunately, nerves to the areola and nipple were often cut, interfering with messages from the breast to the brain. Women who have had this kind of breast surgery make colostrum and breast milk but the volume of milk produced is usually insufficient. The baby's weight gain must be monitored closely. It may be possible to combine breastfeeding with a supplemental feeding system. Newer surgical procedures leave breast tissue and structures underneath the areola and nipple intact. Breast augmentation procedures may or may not affect the supply of breast milk.

Method of Infant Feeding and the Breast Examination

Clinicians often take advantage of the breast examination to ask a woman if she plans to breastfeed. If only the nutritive properties of breast milk are taken into consideration, breast milk truly is the best food for the baby. However, breastfeeding has many dimensions for women in the United States.

Most important may be a woman's subjective feelings about this activity. Some women are uncomfortable with the idea of breastfeeding, perceiving it to be embarrassing, painful, inconvenient, energy draining, and time consuming. Some believe they will never have a chance to get away from the baby, or that their partner will be deprived of an opportunity to participate in a meaningful way in the baby's care. Some women see bottle feeding as a status symbol or, because they will be returning to work, feel they should just go ahead and start with the bottle. Some women may have experienced sexual abuse involving their breasts. Some may have had friends who tried to breastfeed with cracked and bleeding nipples, or may be living a chaotic life that allows no time to sit and feed a baby.

What should clinicians do when confronted with a woman who is reluctant or unwilling to try breastfeeding, when all the evidence favors breast milk for every baby? Find out the mother's reason for bottle feeding. If a previous breastfeeding experience was unsuccessful, it is easy to understand her reluctance to try again. Her lack of success may be in direct proportion to the support and help she received in the initial days of nursing. *If supportive and readily available assistance can be guaranteed,* it may be appropriate to discuss another attempt at breastfeeding.

Correcting misinformation may also be helpful. After that, acknowledging that the client is best equipped to make the best decision for herself and her baby in regard to breastfeeding, and accepting this decision, is the best action to take. Pushing a woman to breastfeed when she does not wish to do so rarely results in a successful breastfeeding experience. Emphasizing the benefits of breastfeeding while devaluing a woman's personal reasons for not wanting to nurse her baby can cause the client to have feelings of guilt that are neither fitting nor helpful. A supportive, considerate response to a woman's desire to bottle feed her baby, combined with thoughtful, attentive prenatal and postpartum care, may make the client willing to try breastfeeding should she become pregnant again.

Consider asking "How do you plan to feed your baby?" rather than "Are you going to breastfeed?" Choose a time other than during the breast examination to make this inquiry. Women who have had sexual abuse involving their breasts may become anxious when they are examined. Asking permission to conduct this part of the examination is often appreciated.

Examination of the Abdomen

Examination of the abdomen in the first half of pregnancy should be as thorough as the enlarged uterus permits. Evaluate for tenderness, masses, hernias, and enlargement of liver, spleen, and lymph nodes. As pregnancy progresses it becomes increasingly difficult to feel anything other than the uterus. Special abdominal considerations in the pregnant woman include fetal heart tones, the height of the uterine fundus, and the presenting part of the baby.

Fetal Heart Tones

Once the client reaches 10 weeks' gestation, listening to fetal heart tones (FHTs) is an important part of prenatal care. This is the approximate gestation at which FHTs can be heard with a Doppler listening device.

To hear the baby's heartbeat, exert a little pressure as you place the instrument immediately above the pubic symphysis. Slowly rotate it 360 degrees until the beat is heard. If you hear nothing, move the instrument 1 cm at a time up toward the umbilicus until you are halfway between the symphysis and the umbilicus. If you have not yet heard the heartbeat, move 1 cm to either side of midline and proceed back down toward the symphysis (Figure 2-1). If FHTs are still not heard, do the same on the opposite side. Be sure to rotate the instrument at each new position, as it must be directed at the baby's heart valves. If no FHTs are heard with this instrument by 13 weeks, request a sonogram.

While it is possible to use the Doppler instrument for locating FHTs at any time in pregnancy, knowing how to use a fetoscope is an important skill because hearing FHTs with a fetoscope can support an EDD determined by LMP when clients have not had a sonogram. FHTs can first be heard by most people with a fetoscope between 17 and 20 weeks' gestation. They are heard best when the tubing on the fetoscope is no longer than 10 inches. The fetoscope has a metal headpiece that should be placed against your forehead. (Metal against bone helps conduct sound.) Some practitioners use the fetoscope without placing the headpiece against their forehead. This may work late in pregnancy when the uterus is thin, but you are not likely to hear FHTs in the midtrimester of pregnancy unless the metal piece is used as intended. When listening for early FHTs with a fetoscope, be sure that the room is quiet. You may need to turn off air conditioners, and it may help to have the client empty her bladder.

Finding FHTs with a fetoscope for the first time can be helpful for dating purposes if the FHTs are heard between 18 and 20 weeks' gestation. Be sure to chart what you did or did not hear with a fetoscope when listening for early-fetoscope FHTs (+FS or −FS).

▶ **HELPFUL HINT**

If you search and search, yet do not hear with the fetoscope at 18–20 weeks, use a Doppler to identify the location of the heartbeat, then place the fetoscope at that spot.

Fundal Height

The abdominal examination includes making a subjective assessment of uterine size in the first trimester of pregnancy, relating the uterine fundus to the umbilicus in the second trimester, and measuring fundal height with a centimeter

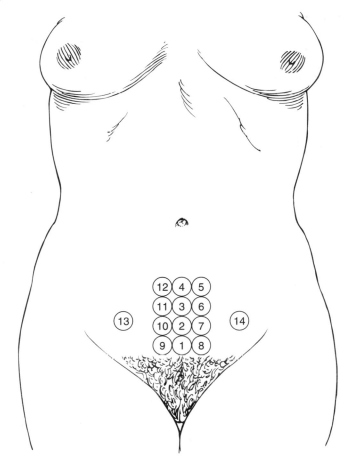

FIGURE 2-1. Finding fetal heart tones with a Doppler instrument in early pregnancy.

tape in the last trimester. In the first trimester, guidelines for gestational age suggest the uterus should be the size of a tennis ball at 8 weeks, an orange at 10 weeks, and a grapefruit at 12 weeks.

Second trimester guidelines suggest that the top of the uterus should be

3 to 4 fingerbreadths (FB) below the umbilicus at 16 weeks;
1 to 2 FB below at 18 weeks;
at the umbilicus at 20 weeks;
1 to 2 FB above the umbilicus at 22 weeks; and
3 to 4 FB above at 24 weeks.

Some practitioners start measuring fundal height with a centimeter tape at 16 weeks. At 16 weeks the cm measurement is less important than growth from one prenatal visit to the next, since it is common at that time for the cm measurement to be considerably greater than the gestational age.

Presentation

An abdominal examination to determine fetal presentation should begin at 28 weeks' gestation. If you are uncertain of fetal presentation late in pregnancy, a vaginal examination may help you. If suture lines on the fetal head can be felt with the examining fingers, the presentation is vertex. Be careful, however, because sometimes the crease in the baby's buttocks can be mistaken for a suture line. Feeling a fontanel makes you certain that the baby's head is "down."

Examination of the Extremities

Examination of the extremities should include an assessment of deep tendon reflexes, examination of the legs for edema and varicose veins, and examination of the hands and feet for size, shape, and placement of the fingers and toes. Abnormalities may suggest a genetic disorder.

Hyperreflexia is a common finding. It should be noted on the medical record so that the clinician will know what is normal for the client. Many clinicians think of hyperreflexia as a sign of preeclampsia. However, "Changes, or lack of changes, in deep tendon reflexes are not part of the diagnosis of preeclampsia" (Roberts, 1994, p. 809). The belief that increased deep tendon reflexes are associated with preeclampsia may come from the days when laboring women receiving magnesium sulfate were evaluated for magnesium toxicity by checking for the absence of reflexes. If preeclampsia develops, any hyperreflexia can be evaluated with appropriate consideration given to the baseline finding.

The Pelvic Examination

The final part of the physical examination is the pelvic examination. Although most practitioners have strong feelings about how to perform this examination, there is no "right" way. While one practitioner may feel it essential to warn the client that the examination is about to begin by touching the back of the client's thigh first, another equally sensitive practitioner may begin by merely informing the client that her genital area will be examined. The best approach seems to be one that works well for both client and provider and gives the client the feeling that she is in control. In this regard, assure the client that you will stop at any time she wishes you to do so.

> ▶ **HELPFUL HINT**
>
> Some clinicians begin by asking the client about her preferences in regard to the examination. You might ask "Is there anything you would like me to know? Is there anything in particular that you want checked out?" and "Would you like me to do this examination slowly, explaining to you what I am doing, or would you like me to do it as quickly as possible so that it will be over?"

Unless the client wants the examination over with as soon as possible, explain that the examination has three parts: inspection of the genital area, insertion of the speculum, and examination of the uterus and ovaries with two of the examiner's fingers in the vagina and her or his hand on the client's abdomen. Tell the client approximately how long the procedure will take. Offer to let her see and feel the speculum.

▶ HELPFUL HINT

Some women appreciate something to hold on to during the pelvic examination. A stuffed animal serves this purpose well. Keep it at the head of the examination table and offer it to all women. (From Karen Parker, CNM, Portland, OR)

It is nice to offer the client an "educational" pelvic. In this examination a woman is positioned so that she can see her external genitalia by placing a hand mirror between her legs (Figure 2-2). The examiner points out the labia majora, the labia minora, the hymen, vaginal opening, urethra, clitoris, and the perineum. It is often helpful to use both the anatomic name and a name that may be more familiar when doing this. For example, you might say "These are the labia majora, the outer lips, and these are the labia minora, the inner lips."

Avoid the use of the words "large" and "small" when you point out the labia because of the connotation these words may have and because, in some women, the labia majora, the big lips, are smaller than the labia minora, the small lips. Women who are learning about their own anatomy can be reassured that any asymmetry in the labia minora is normal, something that is found in many women, similar to one breast being larger than another. If the client is

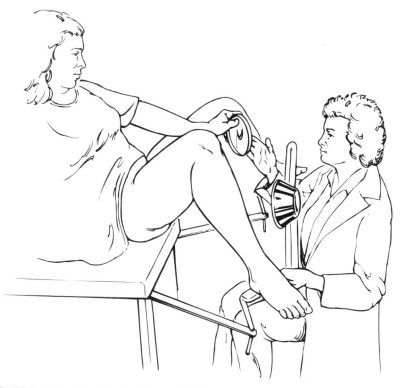

FIGURE 2-2. The educational pelvic examination

particularly anxious, the pelvic examination can usually be deferred for a subsequent visit.

The External Genitalia

Examine the external genitalia by looking for lesions, growths, erythema, discoloration, swelling, excoriation, and bruises. Note any discharge and odor. A thorough examination usually requires separation of the labia minora from the labia majora and gentle retraction of the hood of the clitoris, looking carefully for lesions that might be syphilis or herpes. Be sure that all the movements of your fingers are purposeful. Avoid "fingering" the tissue as this could be interpreted as "sexual."

It is easy to confuse micropapillomatosis with venereal warts.

> *Smaller (micropapillary) condylomata should not be confused with the so-called micropapillomatosis labialis located on the epithelium of both labia minora. Unlike condylomata, in which multiple papillas converge toward a single base, each fingerlike papillomatous projection in micropapillomatosis labialis has its own base. Most clients with micropapillomatosis labialis have no symptoms and have sustained recurrent candidiasis, trichomonas, and chlamydia infections (Ferenczy, 1995, p. 1334).*

At some time you may examine a woman who has undergone a female circumcision procedure. Most of these procedures occur in one of 26 African countries and a few Asian countries, although they also may be done in some immigrant communities in the United States, Canada, Europe, and Australia. Obstetric problems include obstructed labor and perineal tearing; an anterior episiotomy to cut the scar tissue may be necessary at the time a circumcised woman gives birth. The psychological consequences of this procedure have not been well studied. (See Appendix N for more information about female circumcision procedures and the geographic areas where occurrences have been reported.)

Referral to or consultation with a nurse-midwife or physician who has experience assisting at the births of circumcised women can be helpful to anticipate possible problems. Practitioners usually have strong personal feelings about this procedure, called "genital mutilation" by some, and these must be taken into account.

The Vagina and Cervix

After the external genitalia have been examined, insert the speculum. It should be free of lubricant other than water. In fact, a dry speculum can usually be inserted with ease when a woman is pregnant because the amount of vaginal discharge allows for easy entry. If using water for lubrication, use it sparingly to avoid cellular lysis and disruption. Metal speculums should be warmed by keeping them on a heating pad. Some clinicians touch the speculum to the inside of the client's thigh before insertion to let her know what it feels like and to be sure that the temperature is comfortable. Occasionally, the heating pad has been turned on too high and the speculum is hot.

Once the speculum is in place, bring the cervix into view. Remove excess mucus on the cervix. If the baby's weight has caused the body of the uterus to fall forward and the cervical os to move into a posterior location in the vagina, it may be difficult for the client to see the cervical opening. It may also be difficult to obtain specimens for the Pap smear and cervical cultures. Elevating the client's hips by placing a towel under them can make visualization of the cervical os easier. Look for vaginal discharge, mucopurulent cervicitis (a pus-like discharge from the cervix that is usually a sign of chlamydia), and lesions that may be herpes or syphilis. Herpes lesions on the cervix are usually painless.

The client can usually see her vagina and cervix best if she is in an exaggerated semi-Fowler's position or leaning on her left elbow. For the client to see her cervix clearly, the light must be properly placed between the client and the mirror. It may be helpful to have the client or the chaperone shine a flashlight into the mirror.

For many women seeing their cervix is an exciting moment. Other women are "turned off" by the thought of viewing their internal anatomy, and their desire not to participate in the "educational" pelvic examination should be respected.

Obtaining Specimens

The Pap Smear

Appropriate techniques for obtaining specimens for the Pap smear and for gonorrhea and chlamydia testing should be observed. Some clinicians prefer to obtain secretions for the Pap smear first, while others first obtain secretions for gonorrhea and chlamydia testing. Those who recommend obtaining secretions for the Pap smear first know that blood on the slide can affect the interpretation of the specimen. Since the likelihood of bleeding increases with each sample obtained, these clinicians obtain the Pap first.

The real test of the best way to obtain a Pap smear is whether or not the specimens are adequate for interpretation. An optimum specimen for Pap smear interpretation involves the absence of intercourse and douching for 24 hours prior to the test. Clients should be advised of this when they schedule their initial appointment.

Sample both the exocervix and the endocervix for the Pap smear. A brush sampling device is preferred for obtaining the endocervical sample. However, when obtaining a sample from a pregnant woman, a small, cotton-tipped applicator moistened in saline is sometimes used because trauma from the brush may cause the cervix to bleed. Some clinicians feel that the increased bleeding is not significant and recommend either a spatula, a cotton swab, or a brush as safe for use with pregnant women (Foster & Smith, 1996).

The Specimen for Chlamydia

The specimen that will be tested for chlamydia should be obtained from the cervix. If the laboratory procedure involves a DNA probe, a special, dacron-tipped applicator should be used to obtain the specimen.

Research studies have been inconclusive about complications for pregnant women from chlamydia. Some studies suggest that the risk for PTL labor and premature rupture of the membranes is increased, while other studies have not found an increased risk. However, babies born to women with chlamydia infections are known to be at risk for chlamydial conjunctivitis or chlamydial pneumonia (manifested up to 3 months after birth).

The drug of choice to treat chlamydia infections in pregnant women has been erythromycin, but amoxicillin (500 mg po tid for 7 to 10 days) has recently been shown to be as effective and to have fewer gastrointestinal side effects (Turrentine & Newton, 1995). See Box 2-13 for recommendations for treating chlamydia in pregnancy.

Doxycycline, one of the "drugs of choice" for the treatment of chlamydia in *non*pregnant women, is a tetracycline. It generally is avoided in pregnant

**Box 2-13. Recommendations for the Treatment
of Chlamydia During Pregnancy**

Recommended regimens:
Erythromycin base (E-mycin) 500 mg orally 4 times a day for 7 days
or
Amoxicillin 500 mg orally 3 times a day for 7–10 days
Alternative regimens:
Erythromycin base (E-mycin) 250 mg orally 4 times a day for 14 days
or
Erythromycin ethylsuccinate (E.E.S.) 800 mg orally 4 times a day for 7 days
or
Erythromycin ethylsuccinate (E.E.S.) 400 mg orally 4 times a day for
14 days

Note: Because of the risk of drug-related hepatotoxicity, erythromycin estolate is contraindicated during pregnancy.

women because of reports of yellow-brown discoloration of the deciduous
teeth, and acute fatty liver changes in pregnant women with renal insufficiency.
Azithromycin, another "drug of choice" in nonpregnant women, is a new drug.
Experience with pregnant women is limited, and it is not presently recommended during pregnancy; consequently, some practitioners are reluctant to
use it prenatally. Its advantage, however, is that a single oral dose of 1 g is effective, and there are no gastrointestinal side effects. Because of its effectiveness
in a one-time oral dose and the fact that no adverse fetal effects have been attributed to the drug, some practitioners prescribe azithromycin for pregnant
women.

Routine test-of-cure for chlamydia during the immediate posttreatment period is not recommended by the Centers for Disease Control and Prevention
(CDC) because there are no resistant strains of *Chlamydia trachomatis*. However,
an individual woman's history may suggest the need for retesting. Because testing done soon after completion of drug therapy may result in a false positive
test, wait 2 weeks after completion of treatment to perform another test.

The Specimen for Gonorrhea
Babies exposed to gonorrhea may develop ophthalmia neonatorum, an infection of the eyes that, untreated, can lead to blindness. Pregnant women who
have gonorrhea are at risk for preterm delivery and premature rupture of membranes. If the infection is present at delivery, the risk for chorioamnionitis and
postpartum infection is higher than in women without infection.

Neisseria gonorrhae resistance to penicillin mandated new treatment recommendations for this disease in 1993. A single, oral dose of cefixime, 400 mg, is
one of the recommended treatments for gonorrhea in pregnant women. Because drug resistance to cefixime has not been demonstrated, a test-of-cure is
not necessary when using this regimen unless reinfection is suspected. Sexual
contacts within the previous 120 days should be treated presumptively.
Women at risk for gonorrhea and chlamydia should have a repeat test at 36
weeks. See Box 2-14 for recommendations for the treatment of gonorrhea during pregnancy.

> **Box 2-14. Recommendations for the Treatment of Uncomplicated Gonorrhea During Pregnancy**
>
> A single dose of ceftriaxone 125 mg IM *or* cefixime 400 mg orally
> *plus*
> Treatment for chlamydia if chlamydia testing was not done, because up to 40% of persons with gonorrhea are also infected with chlamydia

Bimanual Examination of the Uterus

Once the cervix and vaginal walls are inspected and laboratory specimens obtained, a bimanual examination is performed to estimate uterine size, evaluate the adnexa if the examination is performed in the first trimester, and estimate the length and dilatation of the cervix. If the cervix is 1 cm or less in length, the woman is considered at risk for PTL. She is also at increased risk for PTL if the cervix is dilated before the 28th week or if it is dilated more than 2 cms between 28 and 34 weeks.

Clinical Pelvimetry

Some clinicians evaluate the pelvic bones after the bimanual examination. This procedure is not particularly useful in developed countries where nutrition is good and diseases are not likely to have affected the bony pelvis. A "trial of labor" is almost always indicated regardless of pelvic measurements unless obvious deformities are present or pelvic fracture/surgery has occurred. Still, this procedure is usually taught in educational programs, and textbooks provide directions for obtaining the measurements considered important. Remember that this examination is a subjective one.

One advantage to performing clinical pelvimetry is that it provides an opportunity to reassure a woman about her ability to give birth vaginally. Every woman deserves to be hopeful in this regard. When a woman has what appears to be an adequate or large pelvis, encourage her by saying something like "I think your pelvis is perfect for this baby." Avoid telling a woman she has a "small pelvis." A subjective evaluation of pelvic bone structure rarely allows the clinician to predict with certainty which women will give birth vaginally and which will require surgery. So many factors are out of the clinician's control during labor—the size and position of the baby, the mother's emotional state and energy level—that it seems appropriate to remain optimistic. If a woman asks about the size of her pelvis, remind her that labor is not about pelvic size but about multiple factors, some of which involve decisions that the baby makes. Even a woman with a large pelvis may need a Cesarean delivery if her baby's head assumes an unfavorable position during labor.

▼ Laboratory Tests

Initial laboratory studies for low-risk women usually include the following blood tests: blood type and rhesus (Rh) factor, antibody screen, complete blood count (CBC) or hematocrit, rapid plasma reagin (RPR) or other test for syphilis, rubella titre, hepatitis B surface antigen (HBSAg), and HIV. Many clinicians also request a urine culture. Individual circumstances may require additional testing. As pregnancy advances, additional tests, such as the maternal serum triple screen, are appropriate.

The Rh Factor

Rh is a factor (antigen) on the red blood cells of about 85% of the white population and 93% of the African American population. It has been found on fetal cells as early as 6 weeks after conception. People with the factor are said to be Rh-positive. Those without it are said to be Rh-negative.

At the time of abortion and at the time of delivery, fetal blood, if Rh-positive, may enter the maternal circulation, causing Rh-negative maternal blood to become "sensitized." In this situation, the Rh-negative mother's immune system may produce antibodies against the Rh antigen which can pass from mother to fetus. In rare instances, sensitization will occur before delivery without any external evidence of bleeding.

The Rh factor is determined to identify babies who could be sick or die from Rh disease (hemolytic disease of the newborn), and women who should receive Rh immune globulin (RhIg) to prevent this disease. Rh-affected babies may be mildly, moderately, or severely ill. Newborns in the mild group will have either mild or no anemia. Newborns with moderate disease will have hepatosplenomegaly and moderate anemia with jaundice after birth. Kernicterus may occur and cause mental retardation and even death. Severely affected infants will develop hydrops, often before 30 weeks' gestation. Death can occur in utero. Babies in this group usually require an intrauterine transfusion, as hemoglobin levels are commonly between 4 and 6 g/dL.

The first Rh positive pregnancy is at low risk for sensitization. The risk of Rh sensitization in an Rh-negative woman who has ABO-compatible blood is 8% after the first pregnancy and 16% after the second pregnancy when RhIg is not administered (Bowman, 1978). The percentages will be lower if the mother and baby have an ABO incompatibility because an ABO incompatibility appears to give some protection to the baby against the effects of an Rh incompatibility.

Rh immune globulin, licensed in 1968 and known commercially as RhoGAM, contains antibodies to the Rh factor. The antibodies destroy any Rh-positive fetal cells in the mother's blood and prevent the development of the mother's own antibodies by her immune system. If administered within 72 hours of birth, RhIg has almost eradicated Rh disease in developed countries, preventing the development of antibodies in 98% of the women who would have developed them. Prenatal administration of RhIg to unsensitized Rh-negative women at 28 weeks' gestation is aimed at the 0.2% of Rh-negative women who become sensitized before delivery. RhIg is also administered to Rh-negative women after any prenatal bleeding episode; an abortion, spontaneous or elective; abdominal trauma; and certain obstetric procedures, such as a version late in pregnancy to turn a baby from a breech or transverse to a vertex presentation.

RhIg comes in two dosages: 50 μg and 300 μg. The 50-μg dose will neutralize 5 mL of fetal red cells, and is given to Rh-negative women with an ectopic pregnancy, women undergoing chorionic villus sampling (CVS), and women having a first trimester abortion. (A fetus at 10 or 11 weeks' gestation has less than 5 mL of fetal RBCs.) The 300-μg dose is used with Rh-negative women at 28 weeks' gestation (or later); after an amniocentesis; with an abortion beyond 12 weeks' gestation; and with suspected abruption. It will neutralize 15 mL of fetal red blood cells (RBCs).

There appears to be no harm to either mother or baby from the administration of RhIg. Although it is a blood product, the donated blood is screened and treated for bacteria and HIV. No infectious diseases, including hepatitis and AIDS, have been associated with RhIg. Because RhIg is a blood product, members of certain religious groups may refuse it.

RhIg protection lasts approximately 12 weeks. Since most women deliver after their EDD, it seems sensible to give this product at 29 or 30 weeks' gestation rather than at 28 weeks. However, the study demonstrating the effectiveness of prenatal immune globulin administered it at 28 weeks; therefore, 28 weeks is the standard of care. Since no harm comes from administering RhIg later in pregnancy, it can be given after 28 weeks.

The Antibody Screen

The antibody screen is used to identify women with antibodies dangerous to fetal well-being. These women should not receive RhIg. While Rh disease is primarily responsible for hemolytic disease of the newborn, approximately 2% is a result of rare blood groups. Table 2-1 identifies some of these rare red blood cell antigens and the extent to which each may be a problem for the fetus or newborn. Note that many do not produce hemolytic disease. Use the table to know whether or not a referral to a physician is in order. An Rh-negative woman with a positive antibody screen should be referred for physician follow-up.

TABLE 2-1. Antibodies Causing Hemolytic Disease*

Blood Group System	Antigens Related to Hemolytic Disease	Severity of Hemolytic Disease
CDE	D	Mild to severe
	C	Mild to moderate
	c	Mild to severe
	E	Mild to severe
	e	Mild to moderate
Lewis		Not a proved cause of hemolytic disease of the newborn
I		Not a proved cause of hemolytic disease of the newborn
Kell	K	Mild to severe with hydrops fetalis
	k	Mild to severe
Duffy	Fy^a	Mild to severe with hydrops fetalis
	Fy^b	Not a cause of hemolytic disease of the newborn

(continued)

TABLE 2-1. Antibodies Causing Hemoytic Disease **(Continued)**

Blood Group System	Antigens Related to Hemolytic Disease	Severity of Hemolytic Disease
Kidd	Jk^a	Mild to severe
	Jk^b	Mild to severe
MNSs	M	Mild to severe
	N	Mild
	S	Mild to severe
	s	Mild to severe
Lutheran	Lu^a	Mild
	Lu^b	Mild
Diego	Di^a	Mild to severe
	Di^b	Mild to severe
Xg	Xg^a	Mild
P	PP$_1$P^k(Tj^a)	Mild to severe
Public	Yt^a	Moderate to severe
	Yt^b	Mild
	Lan	Mild
	En^a	Moderate
	Ge	Mild
	Jr^a	Mild
	Co^a	Severe
	Co^{a-b-}	Mild
Private antigens	Batty	Mild
	Becker	Mild
	Berrens	Mild
	Evans	Mild
	Gonzales	Mild
	Good	Severe
	Heibel	Moderate
	Hunt	Mild
	Jobbins	Mild
	Radin	Moderate
	Rm	Mild
	Ven	Mild
	Wright^a	Severe
	Wright^b	Mild
	Zd	Moderate

*Note that conditions listed as being "mild" only can be treated like ABO incompatibility. Patients with all other conditions should be monitored as if they were sensitized to D. Reprinted with permission from American College of Obstetricians and Gynecologists: Management of iso-immunization in pregnancy. Technical Bulletin No. 148. Washington, DC, ACOG, ©1990.

The Complete Blood Count (CBC)

Physiologic Anemia

During pregnancy, increases in plasma volume and RBC mass increase maternal blood volume about 45% over nonpregnant levels. However, the increase in red cell volume is less than the increase in plasma volume, and a dilutional anemia occurs. This "physiologic" anemia is easily interpreted as a true anemia. Figure 2-3 illustrates the changes in blood volume during pregnancy.

Tests for Anemia

Some clinics and offices request only a hemoglobin or hematocrit to screen for anemia in pregnant women. When one or both of these measurements is the only value used to screen for anemia in pregnancy, two serious errors may result: treating women without true anemia and not treating women who are truly anemic. Providers may spend unnecessary time counseling women about the value of eating iron-rich foods when this approach is unnecessary and inappropriate for the situation.

Red blood cell indices are an important part of any follow-up of low hemoglobin or hematocrit levels (see Box 1-7 for norms for RBC indices. Figure 2-4A illustrates one approach to an antepartum hematologic assessment). Anemia in pregnancy is usually caused by iron deficiency. The red cells will become microcytic (low MCV) and hypochromic (low MCH). Mild anemia rarely poses a problem for either a pregnant woman or her baby. (Maternal hemoglobin levels are not related to fetal hemoglobin levels.) Anemia can also be caused by a folic acid or vitamin B_{12} deficiency or by one of the thalassemias or stuctural hemoglobinopathies. Figure 2-4B illustrates an approach to be used when the client is of African or Mediterranean descent and the thalassemias must be considered.

The three broad categories of anemia based on RBC indices are microcytic anemia (MCV less than 80 fL), macrocytic anemia (MCV greater than 95 fL), and

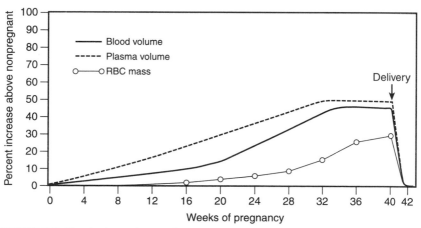

FIGURE 2-3. Blood volume changes in pregnancy.

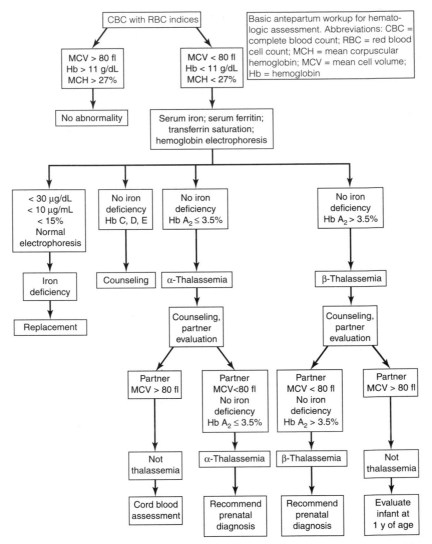

FIGURE 2-4. (A) Antepartum hematologic workup. From American College of Obstetricians and Gynecologists. (1993). Hemoglobinopathies in pregnancy. (ACOG Technical Bulletin Number 185). Washington, DC: American College of Obstetricians and Gynecologists. **(B)** Algorithm for screening for thalassemia when the patient is of African, Asian, or Mediterranean descent.

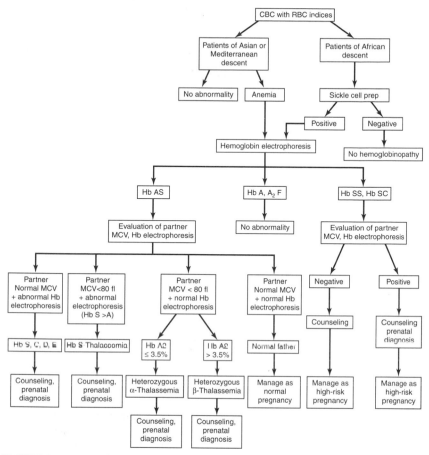

FIGURE 2-4. (continued)

normocytic anemia (MCV 81 to 94 fL). A macrocytic anemia may be due to a B_{12} or folate deficiency, liver disease, or hypothyroidism. Suspect iron deficiency anemia when the ferritin level (a measure of iron stores) falls below 20 ng/mL in a woman with a low hemoglobin or hematocrit. Hemoglobinopathies are common when the MCV is in the 60s.

Routine Iron Supplementation

Official recommendations for the use of oral iron in pregnancy vary. Many clinicians feel that the iron in prenatal tablets is a good safeguard against iron deficiency anemia in pregnancy. However, the U.S. Preventive Services Task Force concluded:

> *There is currently little evidence from published clinical research to suggest that routine iron supplementation during pregnancy is beneficial in improving clinical outcomes for the mother, fetus, or newborn. The evidence is insufficient to rec-*

ommend for or against routine iron supplementation during pregnancy . . . (U.S. Preventive Services Task Force, 1993, p. 2846).

The Institute of Medicine has recommended that healthy pregnant women begin iron supplementation with 30 mg of elemental iron at the 13th week of pregnancy (National Academy of Sciences, 1992). However, it may be prudent to heed the words of an experienced nurse-midwife:

Contrary to timeless teaching, low hemoglobin and hematocrit levels at 28 weeks' gestation do not indicate an increased risk for postpartum hemorrhage; they do suggest, however, that there is adequate volume expansion to tolerate delivery blood loss. Healthy pregnant women do not need another reason to feel that they are deficient, sick, or negligent in their eating habits. This is especially true when the lab test really illustrates a normal response to pregnancy (Long, 1995, p. 38).

Iron Deficiency Anemia

The only point of agreement in the treatment of iron deficiency anemia may be that oral iron preparations are indicated. (Intramuscular iron does not produce a faster response and offers no advantage over oral iron.) Advice varies in regard to the amount of iron to take, what supplements to take with it, whether or not a slow-release preparation is acceptable, and how long to continue therapy.

Recommendations for treating anemia include:

- 60 to 120 mg of elemental iron per day, plus a multivitamin and mineral supplement containing 15 mg of zinc and 2 mg of copper (Institute of Medicine, 1992)
- 200 mg of elemental iron with or without folic acid (Cunningham et al, 1993)
- 60 mg of elemental iron with 500 mg of ascorbic acid 3 times a day (Laros, 1994).

The Institute of Medicine recommends that the supplement contain no more that 250 mg of calcium per dose, and no more than 25 mg of magnesium per dose, since both can interfere with iron absorption (Institute of Medicine, 1992).

The Institute of Medicine also suggests that a slow-release iron preparation be taken with meals if persistent gastrointestinal symptoms are present, but other experts counsel against slow-release products (Cunningham et al, 1993; American Medical Association, 1993). Recommendations for continuing iron therapy after delivery vary from a 30-mg dose of iron for 3 months after delivery to replenish iron stores (National Academy of Sciences, 1992), to 6 months after delivery (Laros, 1994).

Intrauterine growth restriction (IUGR) is not associated with maternal anemia until the maternal hematocrit reaches 24%. In fact, strange as it seems, women with mild anemia have bigger babies than nonanemic women. Why? Perhaps because less viscous blood perfuses the placenta better.

As a clinician, you need to know that

- The amount of elemental iron in iron tablets is usually different than the dose of iron indicated on the label.
- The amount of elemental iron in commonly available iron preparations varies.
- Liquid iron can be prescribed for those who cannot take pills, but these preparations contain alcohol and can stain teeth unless the client places it in the back of her mouth, dilutes it with juice, or brushes her teeth right after ingesting it.

- Iron absorption is greater when the iron is not part of multivitamin supplements containing calcium carbonate and magnesium oxide.
- A response to iron therapy should be seen in 2 to 4 weeks. If no response is seen, a ferritin level may be ordered, if not done previously, to be certain that the anemia is truly caused by iron deficiency.
- Hematocrit may not improve despite iron therapy in the presence of acute or chronic blood loss, parasites, a multiple pregnancy, a folate deficiency, pica, or chronic disease. Think of these possibilities as well as whether the client is taking the medication as prescribed, when no rise in hematocrit occurs.

Thrombocytopenia

Platelets are required for blood clotting. Platelet counts should be above 150,000 per mL, although counts between 100,000 per mL and 150,000 per mL are acceptable as long as a repeat test shows that no platelet destruction is occurring. A low platelet count, thrombocytopenia, is identified more often today than previously because automated cell counters are used for CBCs. These cell counters also count platelets, thereby identifying women with thrombocytopenia who would previously have gone undetected.

The Test for Syphilis

Fetal infection with *Treponema pallidum* can occur at any stage of pregnancy and during any stage of maternal disease. Prenatal screening of pregnant women is the most important factor in identifying babies who are at risk for congenital syphilis. In addition to initial screening, repeat testing at 36 weeks' gestation and during labor is crucial for women in communities or populations with high prevalence rates, as well as for individual women at high risk, because infection can occur between tests. Because it may take weeks for antibody titres to become elevated, infection contracted late in pregnancy can be missed if the screening test is not repeated.

Any woman with a positive screening test should be considered infected until completion of recommended treatment has been documented and monthly antibody titres have declined fourfold by 3 to 6 months after treatment for primary or secondary syphilis, and by 6 to 12 months after therapy for latent syphilis (Reyes & Akhras, 1995). In most cases, once a treponemal test is positive, it remains positive for life regardless of therapy.

The tests commonly performed to screen for syphilis, the RPR (rapid plasma reagin) and the VDRL (Venereal Disease Research Laboratory), are nontreponemal tests. This means that they are not specific for *T. pallidum,* and false positive results from causes not related to syphilis may occur. Accordingly, a positive R.R. or VDRL requires confirmation with a treponemal test such as the fluorescent treponemal antibody absorption (FTA-ABS), which is 90% to 95% sensitive, or the microhemagglutination assay for antibody to *T. pallidum* (MHA-TP), which is 80% to 85% sensitive. If the confirmatory test is negative, the treponemal test result was a false positive. In this instance, a test for antinuclear and anticardiolipin antibodies should be ordered because the false positive test could be due to a connective tissue disorder such as systemic lupus erythematosus. Infectious mononucleosis can also give a false positive result.

Treatment of syphilis during pregnancy depends on the stage of the disease. Box 2-15 outlines the current recommendations. Treatment may trigger a reac-

Box 2-15. Recommendations for the Treatment of Syphilis During Pregnancy

Syphilis Stage	Therapy
Primary, secondary, or early latent	Benzathine penicillin G, 2.4 million units single dose IM (1.2 million units in each buttock). In patients with history of penicillin allergy, confirm allergy by skin testing; if confirmed, desensitize and treat with penicillin.
Late latent, cardiovascular or gummatous disease	Benzathine penicillin G, 2.4 million units IM weekly for 3 weeks
Neurosyphilis	Aqueous penicillin G, 2.4 million units per day IV for 10–14 days
	or
	Aqueous procaine penicillin G, 2.4 million units IM daily, plus probenicid, 500 mg orally 4 times per day, for 10–14 days

From Reyes, M.P., & Akhras, J. (1995). Dealing with maternal and congenital syphilis. *Contemporary OB/GYN, 40,* 52+.

tion (Jarisch-Herxheimer reaction) characterized by headache, muscle aching, rash, and hypotension, that may precipitate preterm labor and fetal distress (Reyes & Akhras, 1995).

The Test for Rubella

The devastating effects of congenital rubella—eye lesions, heart disease, deafness, CNS defects, anemia, hepatitis, pneumonitis, bone defects, and chromosome abnormalities—were first described in the 1940s. These defects are most likely to occur when rubella infection is present in the first trimester. They decrease in frequency as pregnancy advances. By the 16th week of gestation, the likelihood of a teratogenic effect is small.

Women cannot be immunized against rubella in pregnancy because of the theoretical possibility that the live attenuated virus might cause an intrauterine infection in the baby. (No cases of fetal damage have been reported when the vaccine was inadvertently administered during pregnancy.) Women with non-immune rubella titres (less than 1 in 10) should receive rubella vaccine soon after delivery to protect them should they become pregnant again.

The Test for Hepatitis B

Pregnancy rarely alters the course of hepatitis B infection. The concern when a pregnant woman has this disease is that the baby will become infected at delivery and become a chronic carrier at risk for transmitting the disease to others, or that the baby will die of hepatocellular carcinoma, cirrhosis, or both. Infection early in life increases the likelihood of becoming a chronic carrier. "Fewer than 5% of acutely infected adults in the U.S. become chronic carriers, compared with some 25% . . . to 90% . . . of perinatally infected infants" (Oregon Health Division, 1994).

Screening of all pregnant women for hepatitis B is recommended. The screening test commonly used is the hepatitis B surface antigen (HBSAg). Additional testing is needed when the surface antigen is positive, to identify:

- Women who have had hepatitis in the past but are not contagious now
- Women with active disease
- Women who are chronic carriers
- Babies at risk for perinatal transmission of hepatitis B
- Women who should not breastfeed
- Newborns who should receive hepatitis B immune globulin and hepatitis B vaccine
- Families that should be tested, receive immunoprophylaxis, and be instructed in hygienic measures that decrease transmission of the disease.

Liver function studies should also be done when the HBSAg is positive. Commonly ordered are an AST and ALT. Women at high risk for chronic infection include immigrants from Southeast Asia and sub-Saharan Africa. Decisions about which tests to order and how to interpret them are best made in conjunction with a physician.

The Test for Human Immunodeficiency Virus

Whether or not HIV disease is affected by pregnancy is not known. It is known, however, that the virus can be passed from the mother to her baby. While it was once thought that perinatal transmission might be as high as 50%, current research suggests that it is 15% to 30%. A study involving HIV-infected women in Boston, Chicago, Manhattan, Brooklyn, San Juan, and Houston found a transmission rate of 17.7% among infants followed for at least 6 months (Sheon et al, 1996). HIV-positive women who take zidovudine (ZDV) during pregnancy can reduce by two thirds the risk of transmitting the virus to their babies (Connor et al, 1994). Consequently, the U.S. Public Health Service has recommended that all pregnant women be tested for the AIDS virus as early as possible in pregnancy.

Early identification of HIV-positive pregnant women gives women the opportunity to make timely decisions about continuation of the pregnancy and, when a decision is made to continue the pregnancy, to initiate ZDV therapy when it is most likely to reduce fetal infection. Testing also identifies HIV-exposed infants and allows women to make informed decisions about their own high-risk behaviors and available therapy. Decisions about terminating or continuing a pregnancy in the face of HIV disease are complex. Women are entitled to know their options and be supported in their decisions. Information that can help a woman make a decision about continuing the pregnancy includes the nature of HIV disease in infants, adults, and children; the transmission rate; and support that is available now and likely to be available in the future.

Initial laboratory screening usually consists of an enzyme immunoassay (EIA) followed by a confirmatory test, either the Western blot or immunofluorescence assay (IFA). The Western blot is more commonly done. A false-positive result is extremely rare. More likely to occur is an EIA-positive, Western blot indeterminate result. The IFA test results are usually accurate. Liver function studies should be part of the initial laboratory evaluation of an HIV-infected woman.

Women who refuse the HIV test can be helped to assess their risk for having the AIDS virus with the questions in Box 2-16. High-risk, HIV-negative women tested in early pregnancy who do not practice safe sex should be encouraged to be tested again in the third trimester. (CDC, 1995c).

Box 2-16. Questions to Assess Risk for HIV Infection

1. Have you ever had sex with more than two men in 1 year?
2. Do you have more than one partner now?
3. Do you know if your partners have ever:
   a. used recreational drugs?
   b. been in jail?
   c. been diagnosed as HIV-positive?
   d. had sex with someone who was HIV-positive?
   e. had a blood transfusion between 1975 and 1978, or had hemophilia?
4. Have you ever thought that one of your partners might be HIV-positive?
5. Would you know if any of your partners ever had sex with:
   a. a prostitute?
   b. someone who used IV drugs?
   c. both men and women?
6. Have you ever been in a position where you traded sex for drugs, food, money, housing, or anything else?
7. Have you ever had sex when you were high?
8. Ever injected drugs or medicine?
9. Do you have a tattoo?
10. Ever had anal sex ("butt-fuck")?
11. Do you think your current partner(s) might be having sex with someone besides you?
12. Do/does your current partner(s) have any symptoms of an infection: warts, blisters, sores, discharge, painful urination?
13. Have you ever traveled or lived outside of the United States? (Worldwide, women represent about 40% of AIDS victims, and in sub-Saharan Africa more than half of those infected are women. Women from these countries should be considered high-risk.)
14. Do you think it is possible for you to get AIDS? Why?
15. Have you ever been tested for AIDS? If no, have you ever thought about being tested?

Testing for Asymptomatic Bacteriuria

While asymptomatic bacteriuria (ABU) is a common but nonpathologic condition in *non*pregnant women, in pregnant women it can lead to pyelonephritis, an infection that causes significant maternal morbidity and has also been associated with PTL. Treatment of ABU in pregnant women significantly decreases the incidence of acute urinary tract infections (UTIs).

Unfortunately, the best way to identify women with ABU has not been determined. In many practices, a urine culture is performed routinely at the initial prenatal visit. However, the cost of a urine culture is relatively high and, as a result, reagent strip testing (RST) of antenatal urine specimens is sometimes used instead. The leucocyte esterase/nitrite dipstick test has been found to be a useful substitute for the urine culture in populations without a high incidence of ABU (Rouse et al, 1995). In fact, a positive nitrite test correlates with infected

---

Box 2-17A. Common Urinary Pathogens*

Pseudomonas
Staphylococcus saprophyticus
Staphylococcus aureus
Group B streptococcus

---

* A urine culture that reports a number of "mixed gram positive" colonies indicates that the specimen was contaminated with vaginal secretions.

---

urine 90% of the time (Etherington & James, 1993). Urinalysis has not been found to be helpful in detecting UTI (Bachman et al, 1993).

Women with a positive leucocyte esterase/nitrite reagent strip test can be treated for a UTI and their urine can be tested again with a reagent strip after completion of therapy. In this approach the urine is cultured only if the leucocyte esterase/nitrite test is positive after treatment. Another approach is to request a urine culture only when reagent strip testing results are positive, and await results of the culture before initiating treatment.

In practices where a urine culture is ordered to diagnose ABU, a colony count of 100,000 is often used as the criterion for diagnosis and initiating therapy. However, women with urine cultures that grow *klebsiella* and *proteus* should be treated when these organisms are found in any amount; because these organisms usually are not found in a sample of urine from a pregnant woman, their presence in any amount is significant. (See Box 2-17A for common urinary pathogens, and Box 2-17B for common contaminants of a urine specimen.)

Trimethoprim/sulfamethoxazole (Bactrim, Cotrim, Septra) is a useful drug for treating UTIs in pregnancy. However, it should not be used after 36 weeks' gestation because it may compete for bilirubin binding sites and cause jaundice in the newborn. Nitrofurantoin (Macrodantin) is another effective drug even though it is bacteriostatic rather than bactericidal. The usual dose is 100 mg (bid) for 7 to 10 days. Some clinicians avoid prescribing nitrofurantoin for African American women as it can cause acute hemolytic anemia in people with glucose-6-phosphate dehydrogenase deficiency (G6PD), a problem present in approximately 10% of the African American population. This occurrence, however, is rare (Mikhail & Anyaegbunam, 1995). Amoxicillin, 500 mg orally, 3 times daily for 7 to 10 days, is a cheaper and reasonable alternative to nitrofurantoin, although it is not as good for resistant *E. coli*, the most common urinary

---

Box 2-17B. Common Contaminants in a Urine Specimen During Pregnancy*

Diphtheroids
Lactobacilli
Alpha hemolytic strep

---

* No treatment should be instituted.

pathogen during pregnancy. If a pregnant woman has two UTIs during a pregnancy, she should usually take a daily dose of a urinary antiseptic such as nitrofurantoin to prevent another UTI. The dosage in this case is 50 mg per day.

The above regimens reflect traditional approaches to the treatment of uncomplicated, lower UTIs in pregnant women. Short-term therapy with a 3-day course of antibiotics is recommended by some because it seems to provide

> . . . an optimal balance between efficacy and adverse effects when compared with single-dose therapy or treatment for 7 to 10 days. Longer therapy should be reserved for women with upper urinary tract infection, diabetes, treatment failure, or known structural abnormalities of the urinary tract (Mikhail & Anyaegbunam, 1995, p. 676).

Some clinicians would say that every pregnant woman should have a microscopic urinalysis performed, in order to identify women with red blood cells in their urine because red blood cells may indicate urinary tract cancer. However, almost all cases of red blood cells in the urine of pregnant women are attributable to a benign, familial condition that requires no therapy unless the hematocrit is dropping. Clinicians may, therefore, feel that a urinalysis is not cost-effective and refrain from requesting it.

Special Tests and Procedures
Blood Tests

Certain situations require additional blood tests. In addition to the special workup that should be conducted for clients of African, Asian, or Mediterranean descent, other tests that may be indicated by client history or physical examination include a free T_4 if hyperthyroidism is suspected, and a TSH (thyroid-stimulating hormone) for women with suspected hypothyroidism and for women taking thyroid medication.

Testing for Tuberculosis

Women from countries with a high tuberculosis prevalence rate, as well as women associated with groups with a high rate, should receive a PPD (see Box 1-8). Ignore a history of BCG vaccination when interpreting the tuberculin test (Perez-Stable, 1995). The likelihood is that the positive result is due to *Mycobacterium tuberculosis* infection rather than BCG vaccine. Appendix P identifies the criteria for a positive PPD.

Genetic Testing

The risk of a birth defect in any pregnancy is 3% to 5%. When it is determined that a pregnant woman is at increased risk for having a child with a birth defect, she should be offered a referral to a center for genetic counseling.

Genetic counseling is intended to acquaint parents with the medical facts in regard to their risk for having an affected child, the probable course of the disease, how a diagnosis is made, and the management of the disease. This information should be provided in a way that recognizes the special psychosocial needs of clients and their families so that expectant parents can decide whether or not to undergo diagnostic testing. Genetic counseling can provide families with information about inherited and sporadic disorders; birth defects, including those caused by teratogens; and many adult-onset diseases. Prenatal diagnosis usually involves ultrasonography to identify certain structural abnormalities and amniocentesis or CVS to detect certain chromosomal abnormalities, neural tube defects, and other genetic and acquired disorders.

An amniocentesis involves the removal of 20 to 30 mL of amniotic fluid from the amniotic sac via a spinal needle inserted through the maternal abdomen and uterus into the amniotic fluid. The procedure has traditionally been performed between 14 and 20 weeks' gestation. It is preceded or performed concurrently with an ultrasound examination to identify fetal number, confirm or establish gestational age, localize the placenta, and estimate amniotic fluid volume. Risks associated with amniocentesis include infection, bleeding, or, in rare cases, fetal damage.

Chorionic villus sampling, performed between 9½ and 12½ weeks' gestation, involves the insertion of a small plastic catheter, attached to a syringe, through the cervix, with the mother awake and in the lithotomy position. Under continuous ultrasound guidance, the catheter is introduced into the placenta, and chorionic villi from the placenta are aspirated (Figure 2-5). A transabdominal approach may also be used.

Complications from CVS include limb reduction defects (tissue loss from at least one of the four limbs), such as absent fingers and abnormalities of the distal phalanx. These may be related to the time at which the procedure is per-

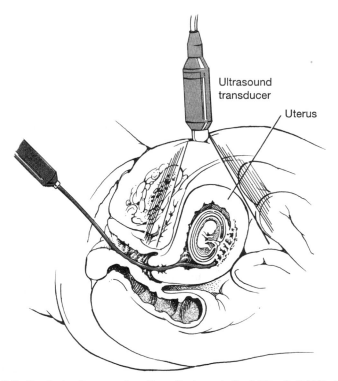

FIGURE 2-5. Chorionic villus sampling. From Shulman, L. P., & Elias, S. (1993). Amniocentesis and chorionic villus sampling. Western Journal of Medicine, 159, 264. Copied with permission.

formed (before 9½ weeks), the instruments used, and the amount of tissue removed. The incidence of these defects vary from one institution to another. Investigations are underway to determine the exact cause of the deformities.

Most of the women who turn to amniocentesis or CVS are women who are older or women who have an abnormal MSAFP. If your client will be aged 35 or more when she *delivers* (34 at some institutions), she should be offered genetic counseling. The risk for delivering a baby with Down syndrome at age 35 is approximately 1 in 370. The risk for delivering a liveborn baby with *any* chromosome abnormality is estimated to be 1 in 200 at this maternal age.

It may be difficult to talk with pregnant women about genetic counseling. The clinician's own feelings about less-than-perfect babies and about abortion can affect a discussion as much as the client's feelings about these issues. Some women feel certain that they will have an abortion if they find out they are carrying an affected baby. Other women are just as certain they would never have an abortion under any circumstances. But time, experience, and information can change people's minds. Therefore, it is important to offer counseling to all women when appropriate, avoid assumptions about what any one woman will choose to do, and support women when their choice is made.

The challenge of conveying accurate, understandable information about genetic problems to non–English-speaking women, women for whom English is a second language, and women with low literacy skills looms large. Be careful about giving printed health education materials to these women, who may obtain little or no meaningful information from the text. Do not use material that has been translated directly from English into another language because direct translations do not usually convey the intended message. Be careful, also, of material written in a foreign language unless you are able to determine that it has been properly evaluated for suitability.

Ultrasound Examinations

In some practices, an ultrasound examination is requested routinely before the 20th week of gestation to date the pregnancy and determine whether or not a multiple gestation is present. Clinicians in other practices prefer to order ultrasound examinations only if an individual situation indicates that it would be appropriate. The optimum time for performing an ultrasound may depend on the reason for requesting the examination. Presently, measurement of the crown-to-rump length of the baby between 7 and 12 weeks' gestation can date the pregnancy within 7 days. Accurate information about dating can be obtained by ultrasound until 20 weeks' gestation.

In addition to dating information, performing the examination at 14 to 16 weeks will pick up almost all twin pregnancies, and performing it at 18 to 20 weeks gives good information about structural abnormalities in the baby. Some clinicians will order sonograms if the mother-to-be is anxious about the baby's well-being or is anxious to know the baby's sex, particularly if they think a mother is at risk for not "bonding" with the baby. Ultrasound examinations are also used to diagnose intrauterine growth restriction (IUGR).

Ultrasound at 11 to 14 weeks can be done to identify nuchal translucency. At this gestational age the fetus has a small, fluid-filled space that separates the muscles at the back of the neck. Increased width of this region (less than 6 mm) has been associated with three serious chromosomal defects—trisomies 13, 18, and 21 (Down syndrome)—and with defects so severe that the infants do not survive after birth. Ultrasound at 11 to 14 weeks cannot rule out Down syn-

---

Box 2-18. Components of a Basic Ultrasound Examination

1. The presence or absence of cardiac activity
2. The number of fetuses
3. The location of the placenta
4. The volume of amniotic fluid
5. An estimate of fetal age
6. The location of the gestational sac and an evaluation of uterus and adnexa when performed in the first trimester
7. Fetal presentation and anatomy survey when performed in the second and third trimesters

---

drome and is not used interchangeably with the "multiple marker screen" or amniocentesis.

Box 2-18 lists the components of a basic ultrasound examination. Clinicians must carefully evaluate sonographic reports. When an ultrasound is ordered for dating purposes, it is easy to concentrate exclusively on that aspect of the report. Be sure that each finding is reviewed.

▼ Health Education

Many clinicians view prenatal visits as an opportune time to provide health education to clients. Four topics are particularly important at the initial visit: signs and symptoms that require notification of the health care provider; what to avoid; what to do in an emergency; and the frequency of subsequent visits. While many other topics could be discussed, confine initial efforts to the most important topics because the time allotted to the first visit, particularly when conducted by a novice practitioner, is significant.

Danger Signs

In the first half of pregnancy women should know to report vaginal bleeding, cramping or contractions, fever above 38°C, persistent vomiting, rupture of membranes, and symptoms of a UTI. These are also reportable in the second half of pregnancy, as are decreased fetal movement and symptoms of preeclampsia. While preeclampsia is common and dangerous, we don't discuss this disease though we should when talking about the complications of pregnancy with new clients. Health care providers need to be diligent about making pregnant women and their families as knowledgeable about preeclamptic signs and symptoms as they are about PTL and fetal movement.

What to Avoid

The list of situations and things to avoid in pregnancy should be reviewed with the mother-to-be:

Alcohol
Recreational and illicit drugs

Dangerous sports
Teratogenic drugs
Environmental toxins
Cat feces
Undercooked meat
Gardening without gloves
Allowing air to be blown into the vagina

The last can cause a fatal air embolus. Since this practice is uncommon, clinicians may feel uncomfortable or embarrassed talking about it, yet it is important information to share. To initiate a discussion about sex, try a variety of approaches until you find one that fits your style. You might say "Most pregnant women have questions about sex while they are pregnant. I wonder if there is anything you would like to ask me?" To her question(s), you could reply "Many people wonder about that," and proceed to provide her with information. You might also offer information by saying something like "Many pregnant women notice a change in their desire for sex when they are pregnant. Has this happened to you?" You could then end this initial discussion of sex in pregnancy by saying "There is one thing I always like to tell pregnant women . . ." and advise the client against allowing air to be blown in her vagina.

What to Do in an Emergency

Inform the client of the procedure to follow if an emergency occurs or contact with the provider is necessary at night, weekends, and holidays. Provide this information in writing.

Frequency of Prenatal Visits

In 1989 the U.S. Public Health Service convened an expert panel to evaluate the content and scheduling of prenatal care. The traditional visit schedule—weekly until 28 weeks, every 2 weeks from 28 to 36 weeks, and monthly thereafter—designed many years ago in an attempt to identify women with preeclampsia, had never been evaluated. Box 2-19 shows the antenatal visit schedule proposed by the expert panel (Public Health Service Expert Panel on Prenatal Care, 1989). Note that the recommendations for nulliparas and multiparas are different.

Clinicians have had varying reactions to the new schedule. Deleting visits makes health care providers who care for socially or emotionally vulnerable women uneasy because vulnerable women often need individualized care. If fewer visits become the norm, these women may be even more at risk. On the other hand, some health care providers like the recommendations because they allow providers to offer fewer visits to women with uncomplicated pregnancies.

Most pregnant women have not heard about the Public Health Service recommendations. If they have had a baby before, they may think care is inadequate if you suggest a longer interval between visits than they followed previously. Other women like fewer prenatal visits. You might give women with an uncomplicated pregnancy a choice. For example, you could ask a multipara at 30 weeks' gestation "Would you like to come back in 2 weeks, 3 weeks, or 4 weeks?"

If you are using early-fetoscope-FHTs to confirm an EDD established by LMP, be sure that a prenatal visit is scheduled at 18, 19, or 20 weeks' gestation, the most likely times to first hear FHTs with a fetoscope. (Note that this may be

Box 2-19. Prenatal Visit Schedule Recommended by the U.S. Public Health Service

Nulliparas	Multiparas
First visit: 6–8 weeks	First visit: 6–8 weeks
Second visit: Within 4 wks of first	Second visit: 14–16 weeks
Third visit: 14–16 weeks	Third visit: 24–28 weeks
Fourth visit: 24–28 weeks	Fourth visit: 32 weeks
Fifth visit: 32 weeks	Fifth visit: 35 weeks
Sixth visit: 36 weeks	Sixth visit: 39 weeks
Seventh visit: 38 weeks	Seventh visit: 41 weeks
Eighth visit: 40 weeks	
Ninth visit: 41 weeks	

From Public Health Service Expert Panel on the Content of Prenatal Care. (1989). *Caring for our future: The content of prenatal care.* Washington, D.C.: Department of Health and Human Services. (NIH Publication No. 90-3182.)

an exception to both the traditional revisit schedule and the PHS recommendations.) If the visit is scheduled at 18 weeks and FHTs are not heard, schedule the next visit 2 weeks later (20 weeks). If the client is seen at 19 weeks and FHTs are not heard, schedule a visit 1 week later.

▼ Conclusion

The initial prenatal visit is a time to learn about the woman who is seeking prenatal care. It is a time to establish a climate of friendliness and concern that will make her want to return for guidance, encouragement, and for monitoring her well-being and that of her baby.

3

The Prenatal Revisit

The prenatal revisit is a time to renew the bond established with the client at the initial visit, evaluate the data that has been gathered, and determine whether or not the pregnancy is progressing normally. Beginning practitioners will find that a considerable amount of time is required to adequately prepare for a return prenatal visit. Do not compare yourself with experienced practitioners who may be able to review charts quickly or even walk into a client's room without having reviewed the chart at all. It is more important to develop a habit of systematically reviewing information and establishing a complete data base than to work rapidly.

Here are some steps to follow to prepare yourself to meet the client.

▼ Preparation for the Return Prenatal Visit

Have a blank piece of paper at your side. Jot down the information you wish to pursue. Whenever you have a question about any data, write the question down. It may be that further review of the chart answers your question. When this happens, scratch the question off your list.

Note demographic information.

Review the obstetric data. What information puts the client at risk? Has this information been placed on a problem list? What information is missing?

Review the medical history and the family history. What information is missing or needs follow-up? What information puts the client at risk? Have all pertinent laboratory tests been ordered? Note a history of any type of physical, emotional, or sexual abuse as well as a family history of alcoholism or illicit drug use. Questions about *family* drug and alcohol use are important but have not always been asked.

Review the findings from the physical examination. Is there anything that should have received follow-up? If yes, has it been done?

Review the laboratory results. Are all the results within normal limits? Pay particular attention to red blood count (RBC) indices if they are available. Not all clinicians know what to do with these results. Do any tests need follow-up? Have all needed tests been ordered?

Review the dating data and conclusions. Consider *everything:* last menstrual period (LMP); length, frequency, and regularity of cycles; dates of pregnancy tests; use of hormonal contraceptives immediately before or at conception; the gestational age when quickening was reported (usually 18 to 20 weeks with a first baby and 16 to 18 weeks with a subsequent baby); the date the uterus was at the umbilicus (usually at 20 weeks despite the fact that the length of the abdomen can vary by several inches from one woman to another); the date fetal heart tones (FHTs) were heard with a Doppler instrument and with a fetoscope; fundal heights; and sonograms.

Note if the client is involved in a smoking-cessation program. If she is, determine if a smoking cessation protocol is being used. Is the chart "flagged" to indicate that the client is a smoker?

Note the body mass index (BMI). If it has not been determined, use the table to figure it out. What does the client want to gain? What weight-gain recommendations have been made? What nutritional assessment has occurred?

Review the problem list. Are all the problems you have identified listed?

Review the previous progress notes. If time is limited, review the notes from the initial and the last visit. Note the plan identified at the most recent visit.

Review any new test results available since the last visit. When reviewing the sonogram findings, be sure to note fetal growth parameters (do you need to use a fetal growth grid?), location of the placenta, amniotic fluid volume, organs identified as normal or abnormal, recommendations for follow-up testing, and the estimated delivery date (EDD) identified from the sonographic measurements. Remember the rules for changing EDDs. Remember the accuracy with which a sonogram at a given gestational age can pinpoint EDD.

Review "Important Data and Key Moments." This guide summarizes data that should be obtained as well as when to obtain it, and suggests times for introducing health education topics (Table 3-1).

Note today's data. Compare today's blood pressure (BP) with the marker BP used in your setting. Note the gestational age at which this was obtained or whether it is an average BP from the first trimester or the first half of pregnancy. Note also the total weight gain to date, and the gain since the last visit.

▼ Blood Pressure

The blood pressure (BP) problems of pregnancy are divided into three groups: chronic hypertension, transient hypertension, and preeclampsia. The last is also referred to as pregnancy-induced hypertension (PIH). Which term to use depends primarily on the term preferred by a given obstetrics community. Those who prefer retention of the traditional nomenclature ("preeclampsia") believe this word better reflects the disease process rather than only one of its symptoms.

Chronic Hypertension

Chronic hypertension is defined as a BP of 140/90 before pregnancy or before the 20th week of pregnancy, *or* a BP of 140/90 identified for the first time after the 20th week of pregnancy that persists beyond 6 weeks postpartum. Obviously, the latter definition is not helpful during pregnancy, as it is not possible to wait until the postpartum period ends to decide about the significance of the elevation. Chronic hypertension and preeclampsia may coexist. While mild to moderate chronic hypertension is not likely to pose problems for pregnant women, it can cause intrauterine growth restriction (IUGR) and fetal death. Severe chronic hypertension may require antihypertensive therapy in clients with diastolic BP above 100 mm Hg (American College of Obstetricians and Gynecologists, 1996).

Baseline data that should be obtained when a pregnant woman with known or suspected chronic hypertension is seen for an initial prenatal visit include a complete blood count to determine the platelet level; a blood urea nitrogen (BUN), creatinine, and uric acid to evaluate kidney function; and a 24-hour urine specimen to determine if excessive protein is being excreted by the kidneys. Special tests to assess fetal well-being are often begun early in the third trimester. Women with chronic hypertension are best followed by an obstetrician or perinatologist, when possible. If preeclampsia is not present, induction before term is not usually indicated unless the baby is not growing well.

TABLE 3-1. Important Data and Key Moments in Prenatal Care

	Objective Data	Emotional Assessment	Laboratory	Health Education
First Visit	Accurate BP Cervical length and dilatation Size/dates Body Mass Index Genetic problems	Feelings re this preg, previous birth/losses Stressors Support system Need for referral: Counseling, food, shelter, genetics, etc.	Consider: HIV PPD Sonogram Glucose screen	Danger signs What to avoid Weight gain records Books/classes
16 to 19 weeks			MSAFP (15–20 wks.) Amniocentesis	Anticipate body changes and fetal movement. Document quickening Parenting: Own childhood, fears and need for help
20 weeks	FHT with FS Weight gain	Stressors Body image		S/S of PTL Fetal movement parameters
24 to 26 weeks	Cervix check if hx of PTL or if first baby	Dreams Fears		S/S of preeclampsia Expectations about labor Childbirth classes
28 weeks	Weight gain Review dating	Body image Stressors	Glu screen Rh immune globulin	
36 weeks	Presentation	Labor fears	Consider repeating: Hct. GC and chlamydia RPR, HIV, HbsAg Schedule version if breech	Prepare for baby Review S/S of labor and preeclampsia Sibling preparation Birth planning meeting

Transient Hypertension

Transient hypertension usually is defined as hypertension that develops late in pregnancy or in the first 24 hours postpartum, without other signs of preeclampsia or preexisting hypertension. It usually develops around 38 weeks' gestation and may be an early sign of preeclampsia or unrecognized chronic hypertension (Sibai, 1996). If the preeclamptic laboratory test results (blood and urine) are normal, the baby is growing well, and the amount of amniotic fluid is within the normal range, prenatal visits and checking of urine with a reagent strip for protein should occur twice weekly. Tests of fetal well-being usually are not indicated.

Preeclampsia

Preeclampsia is a complex disease. In its extreme form it affects the liver, kidneys, central nervous system, and blood coagulation mechanism, and may cause maternal convulsions (eclampsia), intracranial hemorrhage, pulmonary edema, and clotting disorders. Preeclampsia occurs most frequently in women with one of the following circumstances:

Experiencing a first pregnancy
Carrying more than one fetus
Pregnant by a new sexual partner
Chronic hypertension, diabetes, or obesity
A mother or sister who has been eclamptic or severely preeclamptic
Age younger or older than usual. The age curve for risk is J-shaped.

The fundamental cause is unknown, and progression of the disease is poorly understood. Research indicates that the source of the problem probably lies in the placenta. For some reason the placenta becomes hypoxic early in pregnancy and releases toxins which damage the endothelial cells that line the blood vessels. This allows fluid to leave the intravascular space, and activates coagulation factors which decrease platelets and expose the smooth muscle of the arteries to vasoactive substances, resulting in vasospasm and hypertension.

A triad of signs—elevated BP, proteinuria, and edema—occurring between the 20th week of pregnancy and the 14th postpartum day, is used to make a diagnosis. Significant BP is defined as a systolic reading at or greater than 140 mm Hg, or a diastolic reading at or greater than 90 mm Hg. For many years, an increase in BP of 30 mm Hg systolic or 15 mm Hg diastolic from second-trimester values was also considered diagnostic when proteinuria and/or edema were also present. "This concept is no longer considered valid" (American College of Obstetricians and Gynecologists, 1996, p. 2).

Some clinicians feel that hyperreflexia contributes to the diagnosis. "However, the degree of hyperreflexia has not been shown to correlate with the severity of the disease process. The presence or absence of hyperreflexia should not be a factor in making or excluding the diagnosis of PIH" (American College of Ostetricians and Gynecologists, 1996, p. 3).

When preeclampsia is suspected, blood and urine tests are frequently performed to support the diagnosis. Unfortunately, there is wide variation in the use of these tests as well as in the norms that define abnormality. Tests commonly requested are uric acid to assess kidney involvement, aspartate aminotransferase (AST) to assess liver involvement, and a platelet count to identify potential clotting problems. Other tests ordered may be a BUN and creatinine for additional information about kidney involvement, and a hematocrit to identify the extent of hemoconcentration. Normal pregnancy values for these tests can be found in Box 3-1.

Obtaining a 24-hour urine specimen to establish the amount of protein in the urine is essential to help differentiate between preeclampsia and other causes of elevated BP. More than 5 g of protein in 24 hours automatically puts the client in the severe preeclampsia category. Amounts between 300 mg and 5 g are usually associated with mild preeclampsia. Less than 300 mg of protein with normal blood values but an elevated BP usually indicates transient hypertension.

Use of the 24-hour urine specimen to aid in establishing a diagnosis is a departure from use of the traditional urine reagent strip to distinguish between mild and severe preeclampsia. Reagent strip values of 1+ to 2+ were used to diagnose mild preeclampsia; values of 3+ to 4+ were used to diagnose severe preeclampsia. Recent studies have shown that the results obtained from reagent-strip testing for proteinuria are not reliable. In one study, 25% of the women who excreted 5 g or more of protein in a 24-hour urine specimen had reagent-strip values of 1+ or 2+, while only 36% of clients with reagent strip proteinuria ≥3+ excreted 5 g of protein or more in a 24-hour urine specimen. Hour-to-hour variation in the amount of protein excreted in the urine, plus interobserver differences in interpreting reagent-strip results, led these researchers to conclude that ". . . dipstick analysis is an inaccurate test and should not be used as a substitute for 24-hour collections" (Meyer et al, 1994, p. 140).

Women with mild preeclampsia are either treated at home or in the hospital. At-home management usually includes daily monitoring of BP, daily testing of a clean-catch urine specimen with a reagent strip for protein (despite the above findings) if a 24-hour specimen has not been obtained, and decreased activity. The client should be instructed to report any headaches not relieved with rest or acetaminophen, persistent scotoma, epigastric pain, right upper quadrant pain, abdominal pain, nausea or vomiting, and "not feeling right." Blood tests should be repeated every 2 to 3 days. An ultrasound examination is often requested to evaluate fetal growth and the amount of amniotic fluid. While some clinicians feel that tests of fetal well-being should be performed, others feel these are not necessary if the baby is growing appropriately and there is a normal amount of amniotic fluid.

Box 3-1. Normal Laboratory Values for Tests Used in the Evaluation of Patients for Preeclampsia

Uric acid: <5.0 mg/dL at 28 weeks
      <5.4 mg/dL at term
AST: <40 IU/mL
      Mild elevation = 50–200 IU/mL
BUN: <15 mg/dL
Creatinine: <0.8 mg/dL
Platelets: >150,000/cc or 100,000/cc to 150,000/cc if a value obtained prior to the development of signs and symptoms was in the same range
Hematocrit: <38%

Bedrest is often recommended, with an emphasis on the left-lateral position to improve blood flow to the uterus and placenta. With the weight of the baby, amniotic fluid, and blood-filled uterus lifted off the aorta and the vena cava, blood flow from the lower extremities to the maternal heart and, therefore, to the uterus is improved. The purported benefits of bedrest include the reduction of edema, improved fetal growth, and prevention of progression to severe preeclampsia. However, randomized trials to support these outcomes are lacking. In addition, maintaining a side-lying position for extended periods of time can be stressful to the expectant mother and does not make a significant difference in perinatal outcome when *normal fetal growth* is present. This position is probably most useful when the baby is not growing well. While often recommended, increasing the mother's fluid intake and consumption of dietary protein has no effect on either preeclampsia or perinatal outcome.

When mild preeclampsia is diagnosed at term, induction of labor usually is recommended if the fetus is mature (usually at a gestational age of about 37 weeks), because only delivery of the baby permits resolution of the disease process.

Women with severe preeclampsia should always be hospitalized. Fortunately, most cases are mild.

Because preeclampsia is not preventable at the present time, proper respect for signs and symptoms of the disease is essential. Common diagnostic mistakes include:

* Ignoring a BP elevation
* Not testing for proteinuria, or not taking it seriously when it is found
* Misinterpreting the cause of abdominal pain, nausea, vomiting (also symptoms of gallbladder disease and gastroenteritis), and "just not feeling well"
* Failing to look for clotting derangements (Redman & Walker, 1992).

Remember four things about this disease: it is largely silent, it gets progressively worse, it can become fulminating overnight, and it is easy to miss because the symptoms can be so variable.

HELLP (hemolysis, elevated liver enzymes, low platelets) is a form of severe preeclampsia/eclampsia most often seen in a partial form (ie, hemolysis and/or low platelets, and/or elevated liver enzymes). BP is not always elevated, and proteinuria may be minimal. Consequently, any woman in the third trimester who reports epigastric or right upper quadrant pain should be seen immediately. The diagnosis of HELLP is based on laboratory findings. This condition is very serious and requires hospitalization.

Table 3-2 summarizes common findings about the hypertensive disorders of pregnancy.

▼ Weight Gain

Poor weight gain may be due to lack of appetite, nausea and vomiting, illness, alcohol or drug use, insufficient resources to buy or find food, an eating disorder, or poor fetal growth. Although women may lose weight when nausea and vomiting occur in the first trimester, loss of weight or minimal gain subsequently, particularly after 28 weeks' gestation, should cause the clinician to look carefully at fetal growth. Poor weight gain is particularly significant in underweight women. Failure to gain at least 10 pounds by 20 weeks' gestation requires a thoughtful assessment of fetal growth. An ultrasound examination may be indicated to rule out IUGR.

TABLE 3-2. Hypertensive Disorders of Pregnancy

Clinical Finding	Chronic Hypertension	Gestational Hypertension	Preeclampsia
Time of onset of hypertension	<20 weeks of gestation	Usually in third trimester	≥20 weeks of gestation
Degree of hypertension	Mild or severe	Mild	Mild or severe
Proteinuria*	Absent	Absent	Usually present
Serum urate >5.5 mg/dL (0.33 mmol/liter)	Rare	Absent	Present in almost all cases
Hemoconcentration	Absent	Absent	Present in severe disease
Thrombocytopenia	Absent	Absent	Present in severe disease
Hepatic dysfunction	Absent	Absent	Present in severe disease

* Defined as ≥1 + by dipstick testing on two occasions or ≥300 mg in a 24-hour urine collection. (Reprinted with permission from Sibai, B.M. (1996). Treatment of hypertension in pregnant women. *New England Journal of Medicine, 335,* 257–265.)

Excessive weight gain is defined as a total weight gain greater than 50 pounds or a weekly gain in the last trimester of more than 2 pounds. A diet history can help the clinician determine whether the increase is due to edema or to calories. Excessive weight gain may be associated with preeclampsia, although weight gains in this instance are likely to be at least 5 pounds in 1 week.

Take the following with you to the examination room:

- Information you jotted down that needs to be obtained, including a list of complaints from the most recent visit, and "Key Moments" items to discuss
- Audiovisual aids you think might be useful
- Stop-smoking questions from a protocol, if applicable
- The "Healthy Pregnancy Questions"

▼ The Healthy Pregnancy Questions

The "Healthy Pregnancy Questions" (Box 3-2) is a series of questions designed for novice practitioners to ask at each prenatal visit, to screen for conditions or situations that can jeopardize the health of the client or her baby. They can help to identify women experiencing the "common discomforts" (CDs) of pregnancy, and recognize women who need information, reassurance and emotional support. Although the CDs of pregnancy are frequently trivialized because they are "normal" happenings during pregnancy, they can cause great distress and can disrupt family life. Relief measures are summarized in Appendix J. Unfortunately, few of these measures have been studied to determine their effectiveness.

Box 3-2. The Healthy Pregnancy Questions

At each visit
   1. Headaches
   2. Scotoma/blurred vision
   3. Nausea and/or vomiting
   4. Pain: chest, abdomen, back, legs
   5. Contractions/cramping/pelvic pressure
   6. Burning with urination/urgency/dysuria
   7. Vaginal bleeding
   8. Vaginal discharge
   9. Skin changes
  10. Fever/exposure to infectious disease
  11. Edema
  12. Numbness/tingling of the hands/wrists
  13. Genital lesions/sores/growths
  14. Trauma
  15. Fetal movement
  16. Medications taken: OTC, prescribed, herbal remedies

Periodically
  17. Appetite, heartburn, constipation, leg cramps, breast tenderness,
       fatigue, faintness, hemorrhoids, varicosities
  18. Cravings (to eat/to smell)
  19. Concerns about sexual activity, desire, comfort
  20. Emotional well-being/relationships/stress/abuse
  21. Sleep/dreams

As indicated by history
  22. Pets
  23. Use of cigarettes
  24. Alcoholic beverages and illicit/recreational drugs

Questions to Ask at Each Visit

Headaches

Most headaches during pregnancy are benign and respond to rest or acetaminophen. Aspirin is not recommended during pregnancy because of potential bleeding problems associated with aspirin's effect on platelets, and ibuprofen may cause premature closure of the ductus arteriosus in the fetus.

While many pregnant women find that migraine headaches occur less frequently, some women experience their first migraine headache during pregnancy. The clinical issue with migraines is how to treat them. The safest approach is to avoid "triggers" and treat with acetaminophen. However, acetaminophen may not relieve the pain, and consultation with a physician can be helpful. A very small number of pregnant women with headaches and a normal physical examination will have intracranial pathology. Only if the headache is severe, constant, unusual, or associated with neurologic signs is there likely to be a problem. Box 3-3 lists questions that may help distinguish between the

Box 3-3. Questions to Ask Pregnant Women About Headaches

1. Is this a new type of headache?
2. How often do they occur?
3. How long do they last?
4. Does anything trigger them? Lights? Sounds? Smells?
5. Do they come on suddenly or gradually?
6. What do they feel like?
7. Where is the pain?
8. Does anything make them worse?
9. Do you have any other symptoms when they occur? Any vomiting?
10. Does anything happen right before you get them?
11. What do you do to relieve the pain? Does it work?
12. What medicines have you taken?
13. Do the headaches interfere with any of your activities?
14. Do you have a history of migraines?
15. What do you think causes them?

more common headaches—tension, migraine, cluster, sinus, and the benign vascular headache of pregnancy.

Headaches during pregnancy can be a symptom of preeclampsia, a disease that occurs only in pregnant women and that, untreated, can lead to maternal convulsions, stroke, blood coagulopathies, and death. Preeclampsia can occur any time after 20 weeks' gestation. The initial sign is usually an elevation of BP. Edema and proteinuria follow. Most cases of preeclampsia are mild, but 1 in 100 first-time mothers will have the severe form, and their life as well as the life of the baby may be in jeopardy. The headache of preeclampsia is unremitting. It is often accompanied by other symptoms—nausea and vomiting, scotoma (spots before the eyes), epigastric pain, and right upper quadrant or generalized abdominal pain (from swelling of the liver capsule, hepatic hemorrhage, or liver rupture).

Scotoma and Blurred Vision

Visual changes, particularly spots or flashing lights in front of the eyes, or blurred vision, can be a sign of preeclampsia or even a brain tumor. These symptoms must always be taken seriously.

Nausea and Vomiting

Between 50% and 80% of pregnant women experience nausea or vomiting in early pregnancy. Why this phenomenon exists is unknown. Attempts to attribute a psychological cause, such as wanting to get rid of the baby, are not valid.

Frequent dietary recommendations to relieve the nausea and vomiting of early pregnancy include eating small amounts of food frequently, eating potato chips and dry crackers, restricting fat, drinking lemonade and various teas, avoiding spicy foods, using vitamin B_6, and delaying vitamin/iron therapy. Fortunately, morning sickness is uncommon beyond the first trimester. Clients often appreciate a list of remedies to try.

Although Bendectin, a drug used to treat morning sickness in the past, was very effective, it was removed from the market because of litigation expenses from claims that the drug was teratogenic. These claims were shown to be unfounded. Some practitioners attempt to replicate the ingredients in Bendectin (10 mg of doxylamine succinate and 10 mg of pyridoxine) by recommending that clients take vitamin B_6 and half of a doxylamine (Unisom) tablet at night. Doxylamine is a nonprescription hypnotic drug.

Pressure bands are also suggested to treat morning sickness. These stretch bracelets, originally marketed for tourists who go deep-sea fishing, are placed over an acupressure point above the wrist. They can be bought at pharmacies, maternity stores, and at some AAA travel stores.

Vomiting that persists throughout the day for an extended period of time and involves significant weight loss (more than 5% of body weight) is termed *hyperemesis gravidarum*. It is often accompanied by dehydration, ketosis, and electrolyte imbalance. Intravenous (IV) fluids are usually required for an outpatient or hospitalized patient . If you suspect a diagnosis of hyperemesis, check maternal pulse and skin turgor. Identify dehydration with a reagent stick to test the urine for specific gravity and ketones. Request blood chemistries to identify electrolyte imbalance and to help you decide on appropriate treatment. Ketones of 3+ or 4+ indicate a need for IV fluids. If no urine ketones are present, the vomiting is probably not as severe as it may have sounded. While prochlorperazine (Compazine) or promethazine (Phenergan) suppositories, oral diphenhydramine (Benadryl), and oral or intramuscular hydroxyzine (Vistaril) can be useful, IV metoclopramide (Reglan) and even abortion, in rare cases, may be necessary to control intractable vomiting.

Vomiting in pregnancy is not always caused by pregnancy. A differential diagnosis includes multiple gestation, flu syndrome, food poisoning, appendicitis, bowel obstruction, increased intracranial pressure, malaria, migraines, medication effect or toxicity, drug or alcohol effect, pancreatitis, intestinal parasites, and hepatitis. In rare instances, gestational trophoblastic disease will be found. In this situation, abnormalities of the chorionic villi create a mass of vesicles that fill the uterine cavity. A fetus or embryo may or may not be present.

Chest, Abdominal, Back, or Leg Pain

Various aches and pains occur throughout the body during pregnancy. Occasionally, pain may signal a serious problem. Chest pain may be indicative of a pulmonary embolus, a heart attack, or preeclampsia. Abdominal pain may be indicative of appendicitis, pancreatitis, gall bladder disease, gastroenteritis, colitis, constipation, diverticulitis, ovarian cyst, peptic ulcer, and intestinal obstruction. During pregnancy, abdominal pain may also indicate preeclampsia, premature labor, abruption, degenerating myoma, ectopic pregnancy, pyelonephritis, round ligament pain, ruptured corpus luteum cyst, or a twisted ovary. Leg pain may be due to thrombophlebitis, sciatica, or displacement of the sacroiliac joint. Back pain (pain in the lumbar area with or without radiation to the legs) from a shifting center of gravity should be differentiated from posterior pelvic pain (also called sacroiliac pain, sacroiliac joint syndrome, and pelvic girdle relaxation) and pyelonephritis. Careful questioning of the client can help identify situations requiring consultation with or referral to a physician.

Contractions, Cramping, and Pelvic Pressure

Clients call at various stages of pregnancy to say they are having contractions. The clinician must decide whether or not these are the normal contractions every uterus undergoes during pregnancy or contractions that could be a sign of preterm labor (PTL). Always take reports of premature contractions seriously. They do not have to be painful to be important. Ask about additional, subtle signs of labor: cramping, continuous backache, pelvic pressure, increased vaginal discharge, and blood-stained vaginal discharge. Every client should be instructed to notify the clinician if these symptoms occur.

Contractions rarely are significant if they are more than 10 minutes apart. Consequently, teach clients a "magic number"—6 or more per hour, or approximately every 10 minutes—before 36 weeks' gestation that requires notification of the clinician and a cervical examination to determine dilatation and effacement.

Burning with Urination; Urgency; and Dysuria

Urinary tract infections (UTIs) in pregnancy may lead to pyelonephritis, with its potential for serious maternal morbidity and PTL. Inquire at each visit about urgency, dysuria, and burning with urination. Urinary frequency is not a helpful symptom in the first and third trimesters, as it is a normal accompaniment of pregnancy at that time.

A reagent strip dipped into a clean-catch specimen of urine can help diagnose a UTI. Because of the cost of a urine culture, some clinicians will treat without a culture the first time that a reagent strip is positive for nitrites.

Vaginal Bleeding

Vaginal bleeding can occur at any time in pregnancy. It can be caused by benign conditions such as implantation, cervicitis or cervical polyps, or coitus; or by serious, even life-threatening conditions, such as placenta previa and abruptio placenta.

Vaginal Bleeding in the First Half of Pregnancy

In the first trimester of pregnancy vaginal bleeding can be a sign of impending abortion, an ectopic pregnancy, or a "chronic abruption."

Abortion

The first sign of a spontaneous abortion (SAB) is usually bleeding or cramping. When bleeding and cramping occur at the same time, there is a 50% chance that a miscarriage will occur. Perform a speculum examination. If tissue is seen at or coming from the cervical os, loss of the baby is inevitable. If no tissue has been passed or can be seen at the os, and the gestational age of the fetus is at least 6 weeks, an ultrasound examination will be able to determine if the pregnancy is intact.

If a client reports vaginal bleeding before the 6th gestational week, order a *quantitative* human chorionic gonadotropin (HCG) level (as opposed to a *qualitative* HCG level, which usually will state only that the level is less or more than 25 IU/L). HCG levels rise rapidly after implantation, doubling about every 31 hours, until 9 weeks' gestation, when levels peak at 100,000 IU/L. Repeat the test in 48 to 72 hours, when the HCG level should have doubled if the fetus is still alive.

Women who experience vaginal bleeding may call to report that they have passed tissue at home. If bleeding is not heavy, the client may not need to come to the clinic or office to be seen.

Women who have miscarried should be counseled to report fever, severe cramps, or heavy bleeding. If a missed abortion (the fetus is dead but has not yet been passed) has occurred, many women will want a surgical procedure to remove all tissue from the uterus. In rare instances, retention of a dead fetus for a long period of time (about 4 weeks) can cause blood coagulation problems.

For most women, the appearance of blood at any time during pregnancy is frightening, carrying with it the possibility that the baby will die. When a pregnant woman reports vaginal bleeding early in pregnancy, it may be helpful to acknowledge this fear by asking "Have you thought you might be having a miscarriage?"

Ectopic Pregnancy

Bleeding in early pregnancy may also be due to ectopic pregnancy, a potentially fatal complication of pregnancy. The presenting complaint is usually vaginal bleeding or spotting, or cramping and abdominal pain. Often both are present, along with dizziness. These complaints must always be taken seriously. Ectopic pregnancy should be a concern in all cases of cramping and vaginal bleeding until ultrasound confirms an intrauterine pregnancy.

Because ectopic pregnancy may present without classic symptoms, suspect it whenever a woman in the reproductive years complains of unusual menses, amenorrhea, vaginal bleeding, or pelvic pain. A history of a previous ectopic pregnancy, pelvic inflammatory disease, a bilateral tubal ligation, or an intrauterine device (IUD) should increase one's suspicion. Immediate medical attention is imperative to prevent serious or even catastrophic blood loss.

Women who experience either spontaneous abortion or ectopic pregnancy may fear they will die, because the physical pain may be intense and the blood loss heavy. After the event, family and friends may minimize the loss or remain silent, fearing to inflict emotional pain by discussing the loss of the baby. Whether or not the pregnancy was planned is not helpful in predicting a woman's reaction to her baby's death.

Health care providers can be helpful to the grieving mother by discussing the grieving process and comments she is likely to hear. Tell the mother that the sadness may last a year or even two, and that her partner is likely to experience resolution of the grief before she does. Encourage her to talk about her experience with others. Acknowledgment of the pain experienced may prompt other women to share stories of their own losses. These can help a woman feel that she is not alone. Also important is the provider's continuing expressions of concern as evidenced by periodic phone calls.

Some parents may find it helpful to read *Empty Arms* by Sherokee Ilse (available for about $7.50 from International Childbirth Education Association, 1-800-624-4934). Other helpful books include *Miscarriage* ($3.10); *Miscarriage: A Man's Book* ($3.50); and *No More Baby* by Marilyn Gryte ($3.60), for children. These books are available from Centering Corporation, Box 3367, Omaha, NE, 68104 (402-553-1200).

If no complications have occurred, schedule a return visit in 1 or 2 weeks to assess the client's emotional status, evaluate uterine size, and discuss contraception if it was not initiated earlier.

Gestational Trophoblastic Neoplasia

Gestational trophoblastic neoplasia (GTN) is a term that includes three diagnoses: hydatidiform mole, invasive mole, and choriocarcinoma. Most women with GTN experience first trimester bleeding. Other symptoms include excessive nausea and vomiting, and a discrepancy between uterine size and gestational age. The discrepancy can be either larger or smaller than expected. Larger uterine size is more common. When FHTs are not heard with a Doppler instrument at 12 weeks' gestation, request an ultrasound examination.

Vaginal Bleeding in Later Pregnancy

In the second half of pregnancy, two life-threatening conditions may present with bleeding: placenta previa and abruptio placenta.

Placenta Previa

Placenta previa is a condition in which the placenta implants in varying degrees in the lower uterine segment, below the presenting part of the baby. A total or complete previa covers the entire internal cervical os; a partial previa covers part of the internal os; and a marginal previa means that the edge of the placenta has reached the internal os.

A placenta previa identified incidentally on ultrasound examination in the first trimester is likely to "migrate" away from the cervix toward the uterine fundus as the uterus grows and the placenta is pulled further up into the uterus. In 90% of cases, the previa disappears. When an early sonogram identifies a placenta previa, a repeat sonogram for placental localization is recommended at 26 to 28 weeks' gestation. Women with a placenta previa who have any vaginal bleeding should obtain immediate medical consultation at the first sign of bleeding.

Abruptio Placenta

An abruptio placenta is one in which all or part of the placenta separates from the uterine wall before the baby is born. It can occur in the second or third trimester. In addition to vaginal bleeding, the mother often experiences abdominal pain, a "board-like" abdomen, uterine irritability, tetanic contractions, back pain if the placenta is implanted posteriorly, and hypotension and shock. Fetal bradycardia and fetal death may occur. The separation may be abrupt or occur over a period of weeks. Any indication of abruption requires immediate hospitalization for the well-being of both mother and baby.

All reports of vaginal bleeding should be taken seriously. In the past, speculum and digital vaginal examinations when vaginal bleeding occurred in the second half of pregnancy were not performed, because a complete placenta previa might be disrupted and cause a fatal hemorrhage. Today, many pregnant women have had an ultrasound examination prior to the bleeding episode that identifies the location of the placenta. If this is the case and the placenta was not found near the os, proceed with a speculum examination to confirm that the blood is coming from the cervical os. Look also for tissue at the os. Rule out cervical polyps and cervicitis as causes of bleeding. Inquire about the most recent episode of coitus as the penis thrusting against fragile cervical epithelium may cause bleeding or spotting. When bleeding in the second half of pregnancy occurs, remember to think also of labor.

Speculum and digital examinations can be performed in the presence of vaginal bleeding in the first trimester because the cervix is still long and there is no danger of disturbing the placenta. Women who are Rhesus (RH)-negative should receive Rh immune globulin after any episode of vaginal bleeding from the uterus. Bleeding caused by cervicitis or a cervical polyp does not require this medication.

Vaginal Discharge

An increase in vaginal discharge is common in pregnancy, particularly in the last few weeks when cervical gland activity is high. While usually related to an increase in cervical mucus, increased vaginal discharge may also be a symptom of PTL, a sexually transmitted disease, or cervicitis or vaginitis, and may be confused with ruptured membranes.

Sexually Transmitted Diseases

An increase in vaginal discharge can be a sign of a sexually transmitted disease (STD). It may be appropriate to inquire about a new sexual partner and use of illicit drugs. It is also possible that a sexual partner has had sex with other people. Consider testing for chlamydia and gonorrhea.

Cervicitis and Vaginitis

Vaginal discharge in pregnancy may be a sign of cervicitis or vaginitis, and may be caused by *Trichomonas vaginalis* or bacterial vaginosis (BV). Cervicitis decreases the elasticity of the fetal membranes, thus increasing the chances of their premature rupture. Trichomonal infections cause pruritus, malodorous discharge, dyspareunia, and lower abdominal pain in about half of the women infected with this organism. A frothy gray or yellow-green discharge is frequent. The strawberry-like cervix described in textbooks is seldom seen with the naked eye. Motile trichomonads noted on wet smear make the diagnosis. Clients often appreciate looking under the microscope to see the organism that is causing their misery.

The drug of choice to eradicate trichomonal infections is metronidazole, an FDA Category B drug for pregnant women contraindicated in the first trimester. Many clinicians prescribe metronidazole, 250 mg 3 times daily for 7 days, to treat trichomonal infections after the first trimester, as no other effective agent is available. Clinicians may also prescribe 2 g of metronidazole in a single dose. Sexual partners should be treated. The most common side effects of this drug are minor nausea, epigastric distress, and anorexia. Clients should be advised not to drink alcohol while taking metronidazole because some people will experience abdominal cramps, nausea, vomiting, and flushing.

The use of metronidazole in pregnancy has been questioned because of its teratogenic and oncogenic effect in certain animals. Two recent studies concluded that there does not appear to be an increased teratogenic risk, although the oncogenic risk was not studied (Piper et al, 1993; Burtin et al, 1995).

Bacterial vaginosis is the most common cause of vaginal odor. It probably is caused by the interaction of several species of vaginal bacteria. When it occurs in pregnant women, it may cause spontaneous pregnancy loss before 22 weeks' gestation, preterm premature rupture of membranes, and preterm birth (McGregor et al., 1995). BV is diagnosed when 3 out of 4 of the following are present: a nonirritating, thin, homogenous gray or white discharge; vaginal fluid pH at or greater than 4.5 (determined by touching a swab moistened with the discharge to a pH reagent strip); an amine, "fishy" odor when potassium hydroxide is added to the vaginal secretions; and "clue cells"—epithelial cells with a stippled appearance—found when the discharge is examined microscopically.

Identification of pregnant women with BV and subsequent treatment to reduce the incidence of preterm birth is becoming an important practice See Box 3-4 for treatment recommendations.

Vaginal discharge may also be due to candidiasis. Most candida infections are caused by *Candida albicans*, although *C. tropicalis* and *C. glabrata* are also causative. Typical symptoms include pruritus, dyspareunia, and a thick, white

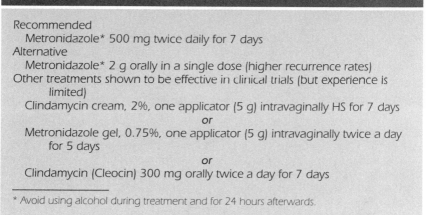

Box 3-4. Recommendations for the Treatment of Bacterial Vaginosis

Recommended
  Metronidazole* 500 mg twice daily for 7 days
Alternative
  Metronidazole* 2 g orally in a single dose (higher recurrence rates)
Other treatments shown to be effective in clinical trials (but experience is limited)
  Clindamycin cream, 2%, one applicator (5 g) intravaginally HS for 7 days
                                    or
  Metronidazole gel, 0.75%, one applicator (5 g) intravaginally twice a day for 5 days
                                    or
  Clindamycin (Cleocin) 300 mg orally twice a day for 7 days

_____

* Avoid using alcohol during treatment and for 24 hours afterwards.

discharge often similar in appearance to cottage cheese. The cervix and walls of the vagina may be covered with the cheesy, white discharge. While diagnosis can often be made by noting hyphae or budding spores on wet smear, absence of these findings does not mean that candida is absent from the vagina. Many practitioners treat on the basis of symptoms alone. Candida infections have not been associated with PTL.

Azole vaginal creams, tablets, and suppositories are very effective in the treatment of candidiasis. These include butoconazole (Femstat), clotrimazole (Mycelex), and miconazole (Monistat). No one brand is significantly more effective than another. During pregnancy the 7-day regimen is usually recommended over the single dose or 3-day regimens. Only nystatin vaginal tablets (Mycostatin), FDA Pregnancy Category A, are recommended for use in the first trimester. However, vaginal tablets appear to be less effective than cream preparations and should be used for 14 days (American Medical Association, 1994).

Oral medications for vaginal candidiasis have not been approved by the FDA for treatment of yeast infections. Some clinicians, however, use oral, single-dose fluconazole (150 mg).

Ruptured Membranes

Whenever rupture of the membranes is a possibility, a sterile speculum examination is necessary to (1) look for amniotic fluid coming from the cervical os or pooling of the fluid in the vagina; (2) obtain a specimen of the suspected liquid for microscopic identification of the characteristic ferning pattern on a glass slide; and (3) test for a basic pH (by touching a pH reagent strip with the secretions).

A sterile, unlubricated speculum is inserted into the vagina, and a sterile cotton swab is used to obtain the secretions. If no obvious "pool" of fluid resembling amniotic fluid is found, asking the client to cough sometimes results in fluid visible at the cervical opening if the membranes are truly ruptured. The reagent strip may also indicate a basic pH because of blood or semen in the secretions. Be sure to ask the client about recent intercourse and vaginal bleeding.

Rupture of membranes in a preterm pregnancy is associated with infection and malpresentation (a situation in which a fetal part other than the baby's head presents over the cervical os) as well as low–birth-weight babies. Clients should be asked to report any leaking of amniotic fluid before the 37th week of pregnancy (preterm, premature rupture of the membranes) to rule out or confirm rupture. **Under no circumstances** should a digital examination of the cervix be performed in the clinic or office unless delivery is imminent, because the chance of uterine infection greatly increases once a digital examination is performed.

Skin Changes

Pregnancy can precipitate a number of skin changes. Those unique to pregnancy that may be bothersome include pruritus gravidarum, pruritic urticarial papules and plaques of pregnancy (PUPPPS), and herpes gestationis.

The initial symptom of pruritus gravidarum, also known as intrahepatic cholestasis of pregnancy, is general body itching. No skin changes are noted except for those caused by scratching. Medical consultation should be obtained when this entity is suspected because medication may be helpful and because of an increased risk for PTL and poor pregnancy outcome.

PUPPPs is a condition in which a pruritic, macular, papular rash appears on the abdomen and sometimes the extremities in the third trimester. No vesicles are present, and pruritus (severe in 80% of the cases) is the only systemic symptom. The lesions begin on the abdomen and usually involve the striae. While topical corticosteroids may be tried initially, referral to a physician for oral corticosteroid therapy is often necessary. Induction of labor at term may be indicated to relieve symptoms.

PUPPPs may be confused with herpes gestationis (HG), a rare skin disorder of pregnancy not related to genital herpes infection. The HG erythematous eruption is followed by papules, vesicles and bullae over the abdomen, buttocks, back, and upper extremities. Malaise, fever, and anorexia may also be present. HG commonly occurs in multiparas, while PUPPPS is more common in women having their first baby. It also is likely to recur, while PUPPPS recurs infrequently. Consultation with a dermatologist is usually necessary.

Fever and Exposure to Infectious Disease

Fever in pregnancy is usually due to flu, sinusitis, or a respiratory infection. While low-grade fevers usually are not significant, a fever above 38°C (100.4°F) poses the possibility of damage to the fetus.

One of the most significant fevers in pregnancy is associated with varicella. Fever combined with shortness of breath may be indicative of varicella pneumonia. If hemoptysis occurs, the maternal death rate can be as high as 50%. Varicella occurring after the 20th week of gestation rarely causes problems for the fetus, unless the mother goes into labor with varicella lesions present during a time period that extends from 5 days before delivery to 2 days after delivery. By the time varicella vesicles appear, the mother is making antibodies that cross the placenta. If delivery occurs around this time, the baby will receive a high viral load, and the mortality rate may be as high as 40%.

Another potentially dangerous virus associated with a low-grade maternal fever is parvovirus B19 (erythema infectiosum, Fifth's Disease). Adenopathy and arthralgias of the large joints are accompanying symptoms. Some women with this disease will also have a diffuse, macular rash known as the "slapped cheek" rash. This disease does not cause birth defects but can cause nonimmune fetal hydrops, an accumulation of serous fluid in body cavities and subcutaneous tissue, 4 to 6 weeks after maternal infection.

This infection is diagnosed by screening for IgG and IgM antibodies against parvovirus. A positive IgG denotes previous infection and immunity against the disease. A positive IgM denotes acute infection, and serial sonograms should be ordered to identify fetal hydrops, which may occur in up to 30% of cases of maternal infection and frequently resolve spontaneously over a 6-week period. Recently, intrauterine transfusion was shown to improve fetal survival after the development of fetal hydrops (Fairley et al, 1995). If both IgG and IgM are negative, mothers should be warned to reduce their risk of exposure to children with erythema infectiosum during epidemic periods.

Table 3-3 summarizes the signs and symptoms, diagnosis, and management of selected infections during pregnancy.

Edema

Almost all pregnant women have edema at some time during their pregnancy. While it occurs primarily in hands and feet, facial edema is also common. Swelling in both normal and preeclamptic pregnancies is caused by movement of fluid from the bloodstream to the interstitial spaces.

Worrisome edema in pregnancy is the kind that comes on suddenly or seems to be excessive. Preeclampsia may be the cause. Ask about accompanying symptoms of preeclampsia: headaches, scotoma, nausea, vomiting, right upper quadrant pain, and abdominal pain. If these are present, obtain immediate physician consultation.

Numbness and Tingling of the Hands and Wrists

Prickly sensations, tingling, numbness, weakness, swelling, stiffness, burning, and pain can occur in the hands and wrists during pregnancy. This phenomenon occurs because the median nerve, which allows movement of the hand and fingers, becomes compressed or trapped in the carpal tunnel, a tunnel formed by the wrist bones, a ligament, and some tendons (Figure 3-1).

Carpal tunnel syndrome usually develops in the third trimester and resolves within 2 weeks' postpartum. It can be mild or severe. In severe cases, nocturnal awakening is common, and clients may not be able to write or hold a cup. Wrist splints may provide some relief. Induction of labor after 37 weeks is occasionally necessary because of extreme discomfort, distress, and disability. *Carpal Tunnel Syndrome*, an inexpensive booklet with an excellent illustration of the anatomy of the carpal tunnel, is useful for client education. (Order from Krames Communication, 1-800-333-3032.)

Genital Lesions, Sores, and Growths

Genital lesions may be caused by the herpes virus, syphilis, or chancroid. All can significantly affect the health and well-being of the baby. Herpes simplex virus type II accounts for 50% to 70% of genital ulcer disease in the United States. Syphilis accounts for 10% to 20%, and chancroid accounts for up to 5% of cases (University of Washington School of Medicine, 1994).

Any report of a genital lesion requires an examination of the genital area. Unfortunately, neither herpes nor syphilis always presents in the classic textbook manner, and as many as 50% of lesions may be misdiagnosed (Hoffman & Schmitz, 1995). Because atypical lesions are common, ". . . all sexually active

(*text continues on page 114*)

TABLE 3-3. Selected Viral Infections in Pregnancy

Disease	Signs & Symptoms	Effects on Fetus	Diagnosis	Prevention	Transmission	Remarks
Parvovirus	Bright red macular rash Erythroderma of face (slapped cheek) Flu-like symptoms Arthralgias Low-grade fever May be none in >50% of adults	Not teratogenic but causes fetal death due to hydrops from anemia caused by erythroid aplasia (RBC fail to mature) Abortion	Ig M specific antibody Ig G antibody titres, with acute and convalescent sera		Horizontally by droplet infection	Risk of fetal death = 9% Infants who survive the severe anemia appear to develop normally Prophylactic immune globulin not recommended.
Cytomegalo virus	15% have mono-like syndrome, fever, sore throat, lymphadenopathy, polyarthritis	At birth, symptomatic: LBW, microcephaly chorioretinitis, developmental delay, MR, sensori neural deficits, hepatosplenomegaly, jaundice, anemia, purpura At birth, asymptomatic: 5–15% with long-term neurologic sequelae later in childhood (usually hearing loss)	Primary infection: 4 × IgG titres in paired acute and convalescent sera measured at the same times		Horizontally by droplet infection and contact with saliva and urine STD Vertically from mother to fetus	30–40% of women with primary infections transmit virus to fetus with 10% symptomatic at birth Acquisition in early pregnancy ↑ severity of infection Recurrent infections = 0.5% to 1% with ↓ severity Seroconversion should be followed by amnio for viral identification

Rubeola	Fever, malaise Koplik spots Cough Photophobia Periorbital edema Rash	↑ Abortion and LBW if maternal measles shortly before birth, ↑ risk of death especially if preterm Not teratogenic	Visual inspection Titres	Passive immu: Immune serum glob, 5 mL IM, within 3 days of exposure. No vaccine during pregnancy	
Listeria (*L. Monocytogenes*: gram pos bacillus)	Febrile illness—may be mild	50% mortality	Blood culture Amniocentesis	Found in soil, water, and sewage, manure contamination, cabbage, pasteurized milk and cheese	Infection similar to group B strep Treat with Amp and Gents or TMS
Rubella	¼–½ of cases are subclinical Viremia precedes S&S by 1 week Only ½ of women with affected infants give hx of rash Termination of pregnancy after 10 wks not recommended as rate of infection and birth defects is lower	If rash appears 12–21 days from LMP, 31% fetal infection; if 3–6 wks from LMP, 100% infection; if 13–14 wks, 54%; if >17 wks, no severe damage but no long-term studies Congenital rubella syndrome: cataracts, glaucoma, patent ductus; microphthalmia; septal defects; deafness; CNS defects; IUGR; TCP and anemia; hepatitis; pneumonitis; bone changes; chromosomal abn. ↑ ab	Visually Titres	Vaccination (MMR)	No fetal damage reported after inadvertent vaccination in pregnancy

(continued)

TABLE 3-3. Selected Viral Infections in Pregnancy **(Continued)**

Disease	Signs & Symptoms	Effects on Fetus	Diagnosis	Prevention	Transmission	Remarks
Varicella	Vesicular rash on trunk, hands, feet, face Fever May develop pneumonia	Early chorioretinitis, cerebral cortical atrophy, hydronephrosis, cutaneous and bony leg defects If delivery occurs while mother has varicella, disseminated viscerd and CNS disease ⅓ of infants with congenital varicella syndrome die in neonatal period and most survivors have serious problems	Visually Titres	VZIG (varicella-zoster immunoglobulin) within 96 hours–125U/10kg IM VZIG to neonate when onset of maternal clinical discharge is within 5 days before delivery or 2 days PP	Transplacental	Risk of congenital varicella syndrome 1.8% if maternal infection in Δ and less than 1% after Δ.

| Toxoplasmosis | Few if any | Chorioretinitis with 50% having several visual impairment if no Rx | Seroconversion from a negative to a positive titre **or** IgM antibodies **or** 4-fold ↑ in specific IgG titre when done at 3-week intervals with no Rx
Amniocentesis
US (hydrocephalous, Intracranial calcifications) | Avoid poorly cooked meat, unwashed vegetables and fruit
Avoid cat feces in garden, litter boxes | Transplacental | 4 out of 1000 susceptible pregnant women will get toxo; if not treated 40% will have an infected baby
Fetal infection ↑ with gest. age (17% at 17–20 wks and 29% after 20 wks) but severity ↓ with gest. age
Treat with antibiotics |

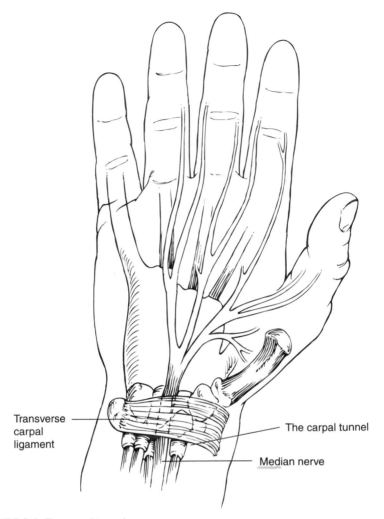

Transverse carpal ligament

The carpal tunnel

Median nerve

FIGURE 3-1. The carpal tunnel.

young adults and teenagers with genital ulcers should be evaluated for both infections, including a serologic test for syphilis and a culture or other lesion test for herpes simplex virus—regardless of the appearance of the lesion" (University of Washington School of Medicine, 1994, p. 2).

Most, but not all, primary herpes infections are associated with fever, dysuria, and enlarged, painful lymph glands. Recurrence varies and is usually preceded by itching, burning, and erythema where the eruption will occur. Obtain the specimen for herpes culture after puncturing an intact vesicle, as dry lesions rarely yield positive findings.

Primary syphilis usually presents with a small macule that turns into a single, painless ulcer (chancre) with well-defined edges on the vulva, anus, or more commonly, the cervix or vagina, where it is harder to see. The inguinal lymph glands will be enlarged. Symptoms of secondary syphilis include condylomata lata (a flat, papular growth on the genitalia), sore throat, musculoskeletal pain, generalized lymphadenopathy, and a generalized maculopapular body rash that can even be seen on the palms of the hands and the soles of the feet. Syphilis rates tend to be high in urban areas where crack cocaine is used and money or drugs exchanged for sex (CDC, 1996).

Trauma

Trauma may result from many activities, including assault, physical or sexual abuse, a motor vehicle accident, falls, and stab or gunshot wounds. Abdominal trauma may be lethal to both mother and baby, because the large amount of blood in the uterus means that uterine injury can lead to exsanguination. Injuries can also cause premature separation of the placenta (abruptio placenta), leading to fetal death and, depending on blood loss, maternal death. Abruptio placenta may occur in 1% to 5% of minor injuries and 20% to 50% of major injuries (Bowen, 1994).

Any woman who has undergone accidental or intentional trauma to the abdomen after 20 weeks' gestation, should be seen on an obstetrics unit to monitor fetal well-being for 4 to 24 hours. Blood tests may need to be performed to determine whether or not there has been fetal bleeding into the maternal circulation. Other clinical findings in cases of trauma not involving the abdomen but requiring hospital evaluation include vaginal bleeding, uterine tenderness, and uterine contractions or irritability.

Fetal Movement

The first movement of the baby in utero that is perceived by the mother is called *quickening*. It occurs between 18 and 20 weeks' gestation in most women having a first baby, and between 16 and 18 weeks' gestation in most women having a subsequent baby.

In the early 1970s, researchers in Israel and England began to study fetal movement. Their hope was to establish a minimum number of movements in a selected time period that would differentiate a fetus in danger of dying from a healthy fetus. The researchers found tremendous variation in movement from one fetus to another. Most fetuses moved hundreds of times each day. However, the researchers also found that decreased fetal movement can be a sign of fetal jeopardy.

A number of protocols to determine fetal movement and forms on which to record daily findings have been devised. Because the number of reassuring movements in a given time period has not been precisely determined, individual practices must decide which guidelines to use.

One approach is to ask a woman to lie down and concentrate on the baby. As soon as the baby has moved 5 times, the counting can stop until the next evaluation period. An accepted guideline for fetal movement is 10 movements in a 12-hour period. If the baby does not move 10 times in 12 hours, a Movement Alarm Signal (MAS) is said to have occurred and the client should notify the health care provider immediately for additional monitoring. Some practices prefer 5 movements in 6 or 10 hours. At times it is difficult to distinguish a sick baby who is not moving from a healthy baby who is sleeping. Normal sleep/wake cycles occur in utero on the average of every 40 minutes in healthy babies.

Women should be taught to count their baby's movements whenever they feel there has been a decrease in the usual pattern. How to count the movement and the form for recording movements should be individualized to the reading level of the client. Lifestyle should also be taken into account. For example, methods that require counting for extended time periods may not be reasonable for women who are employed or distracted by other children. Forms that initiate counting in the morning may not be appropriate for women who work nights. Many charts and forms may not work well for women with low literacy skills, particularly if the chart requires use of a graph.

On rare occasions a baby moves so little that the mother describes fetal movement as absent. While lack of maternal awareness may explain failure to perceive movement at times, reports of absent or decreased movement should always be taken seriously and special testing ordered. Because some women still think it is normal for the baby's movements in utero to slow down before labor begins, be certain that every mother knows this is not so.

Prescription, Over-the-Counter, and Herbal Medicine

Most medicines used appropriately contribute significantly to quality of life, but during pregnancy practitioners must be aware of the FDA category of all medicine prescribed. The clinician is responsible for knowing what medicine, if any, the client is taking; the dosage and the frequency; any side effects the client may be experiencing; and whether the client wants to discontinue the medicine.

Both beginning and experienced practitioners would do well to maintain a system of information that provides pertinent information about the use of drugs in pregnancy and lactation. Any commercially available set of drug cards can serve as a starting point. Discard the cards you are not likely to use, punch holes in the upper left corner of those remaining, and insert them on to a large metal key ring. When you use a drug, read about it extensively (eg, in the AMA's annual *Drug Evaluations*), note the FDA category, call a pharmacy for the price, look in the *Physician's Desk Reference* to see how it is supplied, and add this information to your card.

Prenatal Vitamins

Routine use of prenatal vitamins is not recommended by the Institute of Medicine. These vitamins are big and powerful, and there is no proof that they help women who are at a weight appropriate for their height, eat a well-balanced diet, carry one fetus, and are not abusing drugs, alcohol, or cigarettes. However, a multivitamin and mineral preparation is recommended by the Institute of Medicine when the client

- Has iron-deficiency anemia
- Is a complete vegetarian
- Is carrying more than one baby
- Resists improving a poor-quality diet
- Is a heavy cigarette smoker
- Abuses alcohol
- Is under 25, or
- Is not able to or interested in consuming calcium-rich milk products (National Academy of Science).

Many pregnant women come to their first prenatal visit already taking prenatal vitamins. These women usually do not feel comfortable not taking them, and they probably should not be asked to stop, even when they do not fall into the Institute of Medicine groups for whom supplementation is recommended. It is easy to understand why most women feel that prenatal vitamins are essential in pregnancy. The prenatal vitamin-and-iron ritual has a long tradition. Clinicians themselves find it difficult not to prescribe these vitamins routinely. However, the potential effect of high doses of vitamins is unknown and large doses can mask a vitamin B_{12} deficiency. Megadoses of vitamin A can cause birth defects.

The price of prenatal vitamins varies greatly. There is no evidence that any one brand is more effective than any other.

Folic Acid

Most prenatal vitamins contain between 400 µg and 1 mg of folic acid. Folic acid taken daily during the first 6 weeks of pregnancy can help prevent neural tube defects; it does not prevent these defects when taken later. Folic acid deficiencies are rare. The FDA recently issued a formal proposal to require the addition of folic acid to grain products—enriched flours, breads, rolls, buns, corn grits, corn meal, farina, rice, macaroni, and noodles—beginning in 1998.

Herbal Remedies

Herbs are used by many people. A survey of adults in rural Mississippi showed that three fourths of those surveyed reported using plant-derived remedies in the preceding year. The authors recommended that health care providers ". . . consider the possibility of plant-derived self-treatments among their clients and actively elicit this information when taking a clinical history" (CDC, 1995f).

Some herbal remedies used in pregnancy may be harmful, either because the dosage is unknown or because the herb may be identified incorrectly, contaminated, or adulterated. For example, Paraguay tea, made from the leaves of a holly tree found in Argentina, Brazil, and Paraguay, contains caffeine, theophylline, and a "volatile oil." After recent incidents of anticholinergic syndrome in New York City in persons who had consumed Paraguay teas, tests of samples showed that the tea had been contaminated with belladonna leaves and contained atropine, scopolamine, and hyoscyamine. Investigation revealed that a New York City distributor of South American foods bought the tea directly from farmers. It was shipped in bulk to New York City for packaging (CDC, 1995g).

Jin Bu Huan tablets, a Chinese herbal analgesic, have been known to cause bradycardia and central nervous system and respiratory depression (CDC, 1993b). Jin Bu Huan Hispanic remedies used to treat the digestive problems "azarcon" and "greta," have caused elevated blood lead levels in children. Paylooah (Southeast Asia), used for rash or fever, and surma (India), used as a cosmetic and to improve eyesight, have also been associated with elevated blood lead levels in children (CDC, 1993c).

Be sure to ask your clients about the use of herbs when you inquire about medicines they may have taken since their last visit.

Questions to Ask Periodically

Information about some symptoms, problems, and practices during pregnancy needs to be obtained only at intervals, or as appropriate given the client's history. It is easy to forget to ask about heartburn, constipation, leg cramps, fatigue, and the like because they are common and seem so "ordinary." Yet pregnant women often appreciate the clinician's awareness that these seemingly small things can make aspects of pregnancy unpleasant, if not difficult.

Cravings

Consumption of nonfoods and excessive consumption of some food staples during pregnancy is known as pica, a poorly studied phenomenon that can occur in both pregnant and nonpregnant women. It is associated with iron deficiency anemia and can cause medical complications, with symptoms of pain, nausea, and vomiting (Adler & Olscamp, 1995). Some practitioners who have worked in the southern part of the United States know of a special type of clay from that region which is often shipped to other parts of the country, to be baked and eaten by pregnant women who have a craving for it.

Pregnant women may crave the smell of certain substances as well as food (see Box 3-5). Since women seldom volunteer this information because of feelings of guilt or fear that they have harmed their baby, ask at intervals "Do you ever crave to put something in your mouth or to smell anything? What about cravings for clay, ice, dirt, starch, cornstarch, or anything else?"

Box 3-5. Substances Reported to Have Been Craved by Pregnant Women

Pica Substances Ingested	Pica Substances Chewed and Removed from the Mouth	Olfactory Craving Substances Smelled
Baking powder	Aspirin tablets	Air freshener, scented, aerosol
Baking soda	Concrete chips	Air, freezer and air conditioner
Chalk	Foam of shoulder pads	
Cigarette ashes	Gum	Alcohol, rubbing
Cleanser, powdered	Paper bags, brown	Ammonia, lemon-scented
Detergent, powdered	Paper, writing and note-book	Bleach, liquid
Dirt, from flower pots, ground, out of town	Plastic bag tops, self-closing	Bleach, liquid lemon-scented
Flour	Plastic, of ink pens	Bricks crushed from condemned buildings
Freezer frost	Sponge of hair rollers	Carpet deodorizer, aerosol
Ice, crushed, cubed, chopped	Styrofoam packaging and cups	Chalk
Match tips	Tissues	Cigarettes
Milk, dry powdered	Toilet paper, scented, non-scented, white, colored	Cleaning solution, pine oil
Powder, baby and adult	Toothpicks	Cleanser, powdered
Snow	Wax, Halloween costume	Concrete chips
Toothpaste	Wax, melted candle	Detergent, powdered
		Dirt, wet
		Exhaust, automobile
		Gasoline
		Incense
		Nail polish remover
		Pens, marking
		Powder, baby and adult
		Room disinfectant, aerosol
		Toilet paper, scented

*From Cooksey, N.R. (1995). Pica and olfactory craving of pregnancy: How deep are the secrets? *Birth, 22,* 129–137.

Sexual Activity, Desire, and Comfort

There are generally four reasons to avoid intercourse during pregnancy: lack of desire, vaginal bleeding, ruptured membranes, or labor. Women with a history of PTL are usually asked to avoid intercourse and orgasm from a few weeks before their earliest gestation at delivery until 37 weeks' gestation as well. Orgasm, associated with the release of oxytocin, can induce uterine contractions. Although these contractions usually subside about 30 minutes after orgasm, women who are predisposed to PTL may find that the contractions persist, and may go into labor.

Women (and their partners) often appreciate knowing that a decrease in desire for sex, particularly in the first and third trimesters, is common in pregnancy. In early pregnancy, lack of interest is often due to breast tenderness, fatigue, morning sickness, and urinary frequency. Later in pregnancy, physical aches and a large abdomen may make coitus low on a woman's priority list. Alternate forms of showing affection and, late in pregnancy, alternate coital positions, particularly ones which allow the woman to control the depth and angle of penile thrusting, such as the woman astride, may be helpful.

Women should know that some men experience anxiety about having sexual relations with a woman who is pregnant, especially once the pregnancy begins to show. These men may be fearful of injuring the baby, or they may have personal or culturally derived concerns about having sex at this time. A pregnant woman may be frustrated or confused about a man's reluctance to have intercourse, and may attribute his reticence to her being unattractive because of weight gain, edema, and increased discharge. Women appreciate knowing that the odor of vaginal discharge often changes during pregnancy.

Some women fear that intercourse may be too noisy for the baby. They may be reassured to know that the baby is accustomed to hearing loud noises in the mother's body—liquids entering her stomach, air entering and leaving her lungs, her heartbeat, food moving through the intestines, and urination. Women also can be told fetal movement may occur during sexual activity.

Emotional Well-being, Relationships, Stress, and Abuse

Emotional lability is common during pregnancy. Mood swings may be related to hormones, physical discomfort, changes in body image, or anxiety about the profound way that a baby may affect relationships, lifestyle, and responsibilities. You might say to the client "Most women note some mood swings or changes in their emotions when they are pregnant. I'm wondering if you have noticed anything."

Since stressors and their intensity in a person's life often change during pregnancy, it is also appropriate to ask at intervals about how things are going. You might ask "What is the biggest stress in your life right now?" or "How much stress are you under?" You can use the "1 to 10 scale" and ask "On a scale of 1 to 10, how would you say things are going for you right now?" Women who report high stress, unexplained somatic symptoms, or irritability, alone or in combination, should be screened for depression.

When asking questions about stress, periodically ask about abuse. A review of 13 studies examining the prevalence of violence against pregnant women concluded, ". . . repeated questioning throughout the pregnancy or asking respondents later in pregnancy is likely to elicit higher prevalence estimates" (Gazmararian et al, 1996, p. 1919).

Sleep and Dreams

Sleep is a problem for some pregnant women. Nausea, vomiting, urinary frequency, and breast tenderness often explain why sleep is difficult in early pregnancy. Physical discomfort from fetal movement, a pendulous abdomen, leg cramps, lax joints, heartburn, backache, and nonlabor contractions can make it difficult to get to sleep and stay asleep later in pregnancy. Many women appreciate acknowledgement of their sleep problems and associated fatigue. Problems with sleep can also be a sign of depression, a possibility which should not be ignored.

Unusual dreams can be frequent occurrences for some pregnant women. Common themes include having an abnormal baby and not being a good mother. Women also seem to have recurring vivid images. Ask clients if they are aware of their dreams. Reassure them that dreaming about having an abnormal baby or of placing the baby in jeopardy by poor parenting does not mean that these will occur.

Questions to Ask as Appropriate

Pets

Ask periodically about pets in the home to determine if a kitten or cat has been added to the household. Ask also about the addition of pets that might be harmful to a baby or the addition of many animals that could be too dirty to be safe.

Congenital toxoplasmosis can occur when women acquire primary toxoplasmosis while pregnant. A wide range of findings are found in babies with this disease. Among the most severe effects are convulsions, microcephaly, and hydrocephaly. Toxoplasmosis can also cause abortion, prematurity, and growth retardation.

Fetal infection is more frequent when primary toxoplasmosis occurs in the third trimester, but the severity is highest when maternal infection occurs in the first trimester (Gibbs & Sweet, 1994, p. 690). Many women, particularly those who have had or have a cat as a pet, have protective antibodies and are not at risk for the disease. Testing women for antitoxoplasma IgG antibody is not usually practical as it is often difficult to interpret test results. Women with positive IgG are not at risk.

Undercooked meat is also a source of toxoplasmosis. In fact, infection from eating undercooked meat is much more likely than infection from contact with a cat. Consequently, pregnant women who eat meat should eat well-cooked meat, and should not give undercooked meat to cats.

Use of Cigarettes

Women who smoke should be asked periodically about the number of cigarettes they smoke per day. Flagging the chart with a special sticker to indicate that the client smokes can remind the clinician to ask periodically about smoking habits.

If circumstances do not permit the development of an individualized program for each client who wishes to quit or cut down, a protocol such as that developed by the Smoking Cessation in Pregnancy Demonstration and Research Project of the Colorado Department of Health and the Centers for Disease Control and Prevention, may be helpful, especially when the client is likely to see many different providers. The Colorado protocol involves spending 1 to 3 minutes at each prenatal visit with women who smoke in five activities: assessing the client's smoking since the last visit; discussing the adverse effects of smoking and pregnancy; giving one tip on how to quit; reemphasizing the two best quitting methods (cold turkey and tapering); and providing encouragement.

Ingestion of Alcoholic Beverages and Use of Illicit and Recreational Drugs

At each visit, women who have used alcohol or illicit drugs in the past or during the pregnancy should be asked about continued use. If a special program exists for women abusing these substances, transfer of care may be appropriate. However, women may not want to change their health care provider, and it may be best to ensure ongoing care in a nonspecialized program rather than have the client give up prenatal care altogether.

After a thorough review of the information available to you from the client's record and "Key Moments," you will be ready to conduct your interview. Ask for questions and concerns. Report any pertinent information, such as laboratory results obtained since the last visit. Determine if the client has followed through on any plans made at the last visit—such as obtaining WIC or signing up for childbirth classes. Follow up on complaints identified at the last visit. If a weight gain goal has not been set in conjunction with the client, do it at this visit and record it next to the BMI. Finally, ask any questions you jotted down, as well as the "Healthy Pregnancy Questions." Do not hesitate to pull out the list.

Appendix P summarizes clinician preparation for the return prenatal visit.

Appendix Q gives sample revisit history questions for clients to complete while waiting to be seen, to help the clinician use the time allotted to the visit more productively.

▼ The Physical Examination

Examination of the pregnant woman after the initial visit includes counting FHTs, measuring the height of the fundus, and, after 28 weeks' gestation, determining fetal presentation.

Fetal Heart Tones

Normal FHTs range from 120 to 160 beats per minute (bpm). Listen for at least 30 seconds to increase your chances of detecting any slowing of the heart rate. Short bursts of tachycardia are often associated with fetal activity and are normal. Accelerations returning to baseline can be mistaken for a deceleration. Be sure to listen for at least a full minute in these situations.

A fetal heart rate below 100 bpm is extremely rare. It may indicate a congenital heart block and requires medical consultation. Persistent rates above 180 bpm, as can occur in fetal hydrops, are always serious and require medical consultation. Irregular fetal heart rates are almost always benign but do require consultation. A fetal echocardiogram is often requested.

FHTs are easier to find after 26 weeks' gestation. Listen for them in the middle of either lower quadrant of the abdomen. If FHTs are not found there, listen with the fetoscope placed in the middle of the midline separating these quadrants; place the fetoscope directly on top of the umbilicus; or listen for them in the middle of the upper abdominal quadrants (Figure 3-2). When you find FHTs in one of the upper quadrants, the baby may be in a breech presentation.

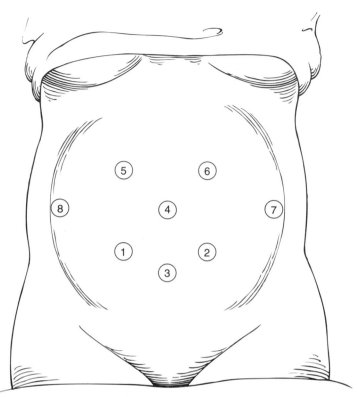

FIGURE 3-2. Finding fetal heart tones after the 26th week of pregnancy.
1 and 2: Listen first in the middle of either of the lower quadrants of the abdomen.
3. If heart tones are not found, listen in the middle of an imaginary line drawn from the umbilicus to the middle of the top of the pubic hair.
4. If not found, listen directly over the umbilicus.
5 and 6. If not yet found, listen in the middle of either of the upper quadrants of the abdomen.
7 and 8. If still not found, listen about 4 inches away from the umbilicus toward the flank.

Some clinicians determine fetal position before looking for FHTs, knowing that it is easiest to hear them through the fetal back. This works well except that babies in utero frequently assume posterior positions, making the back unavailable; clinicians are notoriously wrong in identifying fetal position from abdominal palpation; and moving the fetal head back and forth while trying to determine the location of the back can cause the fetal heart to accelerate above 160 bpm. If this occurs, you will think that the baby is tachycardic, and may order unnecessary fetal well-being studies.

Fundal Height

Measurement of the fundal height with a centimeter tape is a useful but imprecise measurement of fetal growth. The essential parts of the measurement are identifying the top of the symphysis and the top of the fundus. *Feel carefully* for the top of the symphysis, as it can be tender. Since it is the marker for everyone else's measurements, be precise. Its location varies from high to low in different women. It doesn't matter whether you start at the top of the symphysis or at the top of the fundus; do whatever is comfortable for you.

For the sake of consistency, call the top of the fundus the point that would be the top part of an old-fashioned light bulb, where the wattage or brand name would be printed. This means that you will have to go over the top of the uterus and then push down a bit. The fundal height is measured in centimeters (cm).

▶ HELPFUL HINT

When you measure fundal height, turn the cm tape over so that you cannot see the cm markings. Since you know that cm should equal weeks' gestation, it is easy to subconsciously put the tape on the desired marking and delude yourself into thinking the baby is growing appropriately.

▶ SOMETHING FUN

When using disposable measuring tapes to measure the height of the fundus, note the fundal height on the tape at each visit. Keep the tape in the client's record, and give the tape to the new mother at the time of delivery or when she comes for her postpartum examination, so that it can be added to her mementos of the pregnancy.

Guidelines for Growth

Conflicting guidelines exist for interpreting the fundal height measurement. Of the many studies that have tried to determine parameters for distinguishing between normal and abnormal growth, the only conclusion that can be drawn is that the fundal height measurement is inexact.

This is not to say that the measurement is not useful and should be disregarded. Fundal height determinations are widely used in clinical practice, and they serve as a starting point to evaluate fetal growth. Clinicians in a given practice setting should agree on guidelines to identify instances when an ultrasound will be requested to document fetal growth. Between 26 and 36 weeks, a helpful guideline is this: the measurement in cm should equal weeks' gestation, plus or minus 2 cm. For example, if a woman is 28 weeks pregnant, the fundal height should measure between 26 cm and 30 cm.

What guidelines can be helpful after 36 weeks' gestation? A fundal height that continues to increase by 1 cm each week beyond 36 weeks is reassuring (unless, of course, it is way too high). But what about the fundal height that does *not* increase? One possibility, other than a poorly growing baby, is that the baby has descended into the pelvis. An abdominal or vaginal examination to determine the descent of the presenting part may confirm this possibility. Another possibility is that the mother-to-be is carrying her baby in a way that does not allow accurate evaluation by the fundal height measurement. If the client has had a baby before, ask her how much she thinks her baby weighs. Ask also if the fundal height measurement followed a similar pattern previously. Fundal height measurements may be difficult to determine when the client is obese.

If you are unable to assess fetal growth in these situations, it is appropriate to order ultrasound examinations at 28 to 30 weeks' gestation and 34 to 36 weeks' gestation to verify that growth is appropriate.

Size and Date Discrepancies

When the fundal height is 3 to 4 cm less than the gestational age in weeks, the uterus is said to be "small for dates." Possible explanations include intrauterine growth restriction, a transverse presentation, fetal infection, a chromosomal or genetic abnormality, a constitutionally small but healthy baby, descent of the presenting part into the pelvis, a fetal death, or oligohydramnios (a small amount of amniotic fluid). Oligohydramnios, particularly during the second trimester, is associated with increased perinatal morbidity and mortality. It may be caused by rupture of membranes, maternal dehydration, or lack of fetal urine due to fetal renal agenesis or urinary tract obstruction,

When the fundal height in the last trimester of pregnancy is 3 to 4 cm or more greater than the gestational age in weeks, the uterus is said to be "large for dates." Possible explanations include a dating error, a baby that is macrosomic because of maternal diabetes, a multiple gestation, a constitutionally large baby, and polyhydramnios (excess amniotic fluid).

▶ **HELPFUL HINT**

A word about discussing fetal size with mothers: **avoid use of the word "big" whenever you can.** Is there any woman who can respond enthusiastically to the thought of a big baby coming through her vagina? If a pregnant woman has a baby that you think is big and she asks you how much you think the baby weighs, you can either tell her the truth; try to get out of the situation by turning the question around (eg, by asking "What do *you* think the baby weighs?"); or fudge a bit by saying "not too big."

When there is any discrepancy between fundal height and gestational age, the first action should be to review dating parameters carefully. The same examiner should measure fundal height at each visit whenever possible. If the due date is correct, examine all the data available. How much total weight has the mother gained? What is the recent pattern of gain? Is the baby active? What do you estimate the baby to weigh? While fetal weight estimates are particularly inaccurate when precision is most important (ie, when a baby is thought to be larger or smaller than expected for the gestational age), when added to other information available, the estimate of fetal weight may be useful.

Ultrasound for Fetal Growth

A sonogram for fetal growth should be ordered when there is a 4-cm discrepancy between fundal height and gestational age prior to 36 weeks' gestation. Some clinicians feel that a sonogram is appropriate when a 3-cm discrepancy exists. Occasionally, a 2-cm discrepancy requires follow-up, as in a case where the measurement has been 2 cm greater than gestational age and is now 1 cm below, or when slower growth is accompanied by poor maternal weight gain or weight loss.

Transabdominal sonography increasingly is able to predict fetal size with sufficient precision to provide clinically relevant information. Serial ultrasounds, performed 2 to 3 weeks apart, can identify IUGR, a significant cause of neonatal mortality and morbidity, and long-term neurologic and intellectual disabilities. Ultrasound examinations performed to assess fetal growth include measurement of the biparietal diameter (BPD) of the fetal head, head circumference (HC), the length of the femur (FL), the abdominal circumference (AC), the head-to-abdomen ratio (HC/AC), and the femur-to-abdominal circumference ratio (FL/AC). The normal HC/AC is >1.0 before 32 weeks; 1.0 at 32 to 34 weeks; and <1.0 after 34 weeks. The FL/AC provides an estimate of how "scrawny" the fetus is. The measurement should be 22 after 21 weeks. When >23.5, think IUGR.

Because liver growth is curtailed when IUGR is present, abdominal circumference is the best single measurement to assess fetal growth (Burlbaw, 1996). The measurements obtained from an ultrasound examination should be plotted on a fetal growth grid similar to the one in Figure 3-3. IUGR is diagnosed when the ultrasound measurements are less than the 10th percentile or less than the 3rd percentile (two standard deviations from the mean). Institutions vary in the percentiles selected for diagnosis.

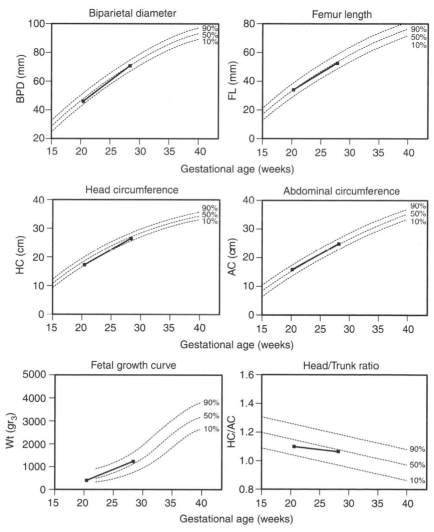

FIGURE 3-3. Fetal growth grid.

IUGR is associated with increased stillbirth; neonatal morbidity as a result of meconium aspiration syndrome, hypoglycemia, and asphyxia; neonatal mortality; and long-term neurologic sequelae. Known causes account for 40% of IUGR (Ghidini, 1996). Often divided into two categories, symmetric and asymmetric, this distinction may be artificial and not as clear cut as originally thought. Symmetric IUGR is said to occur when all body organs are equally small and asymmetrical IUGR occurs when body organs are affected differently. Symmetric IUGR is thought to occur primarily in the first trimester. Since both the head circumference and the abdominal circumference are reduced in symmetrical IUGR, the HC/AC ratio remains normal.

Asymmetric IUGR results when the fetal brain is given preferential treatment over other organs. It probably occurs late in the second trimester or early in the third. Causes are summarized in Box 3-6B. In asymmetric IUGR, the HC/AC ratio is elevated because the head is larger than the body.

A diagnosis of IUGR requires counseling clients to lie in the left lateral recumbent position as much as possible to increase blood flow to the uterus and, thereby, improve fetal oxygenation and nutrition. Clients should also be asked

---

Box 3-6A. Causes of Symmetric IUGR

Genetic
   Low growth potential
   Genetic abnormalities
Congenital abnormalities
   Congenital heart disease
   Central nervous system
   Gastrointestinal
   Musculoskeletal
Intrauterine infection
   Rubella
   Toxoplasmosis
   Cytomegalovirus
Severe malnutrition
   Famine
   Gastric bypass surgery
Maternal habits
   Tobacco
   Drug addiction
   Alcohol
Maternal medications
   Coumadin
   Steroids
Maternal hypoxic disease
   Severe asthma
   Cyanotic congenital heart disease
   High altitudes
   Severe anemia

From Burlbaw, J. (1996). Intrauterine growth restriction. *OB-GYN Ultrasound Today,* 3(1), 30.

Box 3-6B. Causes of Asymmetric IUGR

Maternal vascular disease
  Toxemia
  Chronic hypertension
  Advanced stage diabetes
Multiple gestation
  Discordant twins
  Transfusion syndrome
Placental malformation
  Abnormal insertion
  Hemangioma
  Multiple infarcts

From Burlbaw, J. (1996). Intrauterine growth restriction. *OB-GYN Ultrasound Today,* 3(1), 32.

to drink large quantities of liquids to increase the amount of amniotic fluid. Women who smoke should stop or decrease the number of cigarettes smoked per day. Tests of fetal well-being, usually a nonstress test (NST) and an amniotic fluid index (AFI) twice a week, should be performed. IUGR is most likely occurring in the presence of an elevated HC/AC ratio, decreased amniotic fluid, and an estimated fetal weight below the 10th percentile (Burlbaw, 1996).

Tests of Fetal Well-being

When an ultrasound examination indicates poor fetal growth, special tests for fetal well-being should be requested. Tests commonly used are the NST, the contraction stress test (CST), the AFI, and the biophysical profile (BPP).

The Nonstress Test

The NST evaluates the fetal heart rate without "stressing" the baby with uterine contractions. (Contractions decrease perfusion of the placenta and may cause signs of distress in compromised babies.) While the pregnant woman reclines in a chair or in a semi-Fowler's position in bed, two straps attaching a pressure transducer and an ultrasound device to a fetal monitor are placed across her abdomen. Tracing paper documents the fetal heart rate and any contractions that are present. While contractions are not required for this test, their presence provides additional information about the baby's well-being.

There is variation of opinion regarding criteria that indicate fetal well-being. One approach states that a reassuring test shows evidence of two accelerations of the fetal heart to at least 15 beats above the baseline, lasting at least 15 seconds from the beginning to its end in a 20-minute period; and no decelerations known to suggest fetal compromise. A reassuring NST is termed "reactive" (Figure 3-4A), and a non-reassuring test is termed "nonreactive" (Figure 3-4B.)

The Contraction Stress Test

The CST is similar to the NST except that the fetal heart rate is evaluated under conditions of stress (ie, contractions). If the client is not having spontaneous contractions, they are induced by nipple stimulation or an IV infusion containing oxytocin. A CST often is the preferred test when uteroplacental insufficiency is suspected, as in preeclampsia or chronic maternal disease.

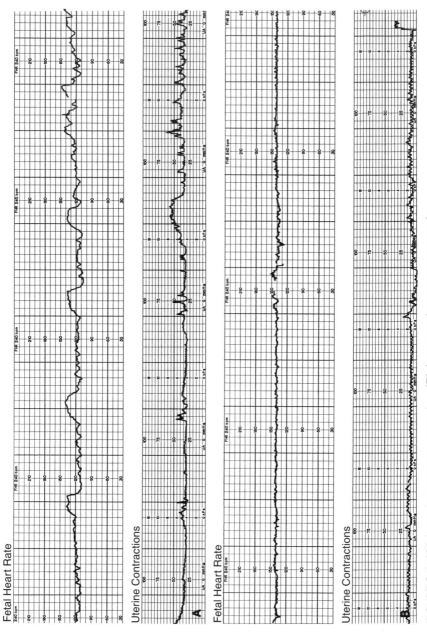

FIGURE 3-4. (A) A reactive nonstress test tracing. **(B)** A non-reactive nonstress test tracing.

Amniotic Fluid Index

The origin of amniotic fluid in early pregnancy is unknown. As pregnancy advances, fetal micturition and fetal swallowing are somehow involved. The amount of fluid ranges from about 30 mL at 10 weeks' gestation to approximately 900 mL at 32 to 35 weeks' gestation. Although there is considerable variation from one woman to another, maximum volume is reached around 34 weeks and begins to decrease around 36 weeks (Figure 3-5) (Brace & Wolff, 1989).

Amniotic fluid provides protection to the fetus when trauma occurs to the maternal abdomen. It also maintains the intrauterine environment at a consistent and normal temperature, and shields the umbilical cord against constriction. The amount of amniotic fluid in the uterine cavity is felt to be a reflection of fetal well-being. When the amount is negligible, the umbilical cord lacks protection against mechanical obstruction that may occur when the baby moves or the uterus contracts.

The amount of amniotic fluid is determined by using ultrasound to measure the largest vertical "pocket" of amniotic fluid in each of four quadrants of the pregnant uterus. The four measurements, in cm, are added together and the total measurement is known as the AFI. Figure 3-6 shows amniotic fluid index values for normal pregnancies.

Oligohydramnios is also diagnosed by an AFI. A total measurement of only 5 cm at term is considered reason for induction of labor. Values between 5 cm and 7 cm fall into a gray zone. A value of 6 cm or 7 cm requires induction

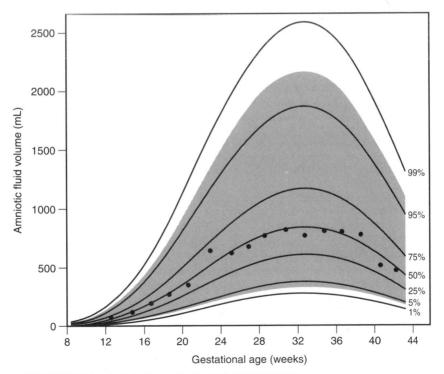

FIGURE 3-5. Amniotic fluid as a function of gestational age.

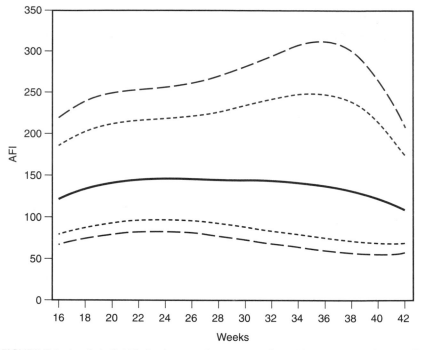

FIGURE 3-6. Amniotic fluid index in normal pregnancy. From Moore, T. K., & Cayle, J. E. (1990). The amniotic fluid index in normal pregnancy. *American Journal of Obstetrics and Gynecology, 162*, 1168.

"soon." A value of 8 cm or more at term does not require intervention unless this measurement is a significant reduction from one obtained previously, as from 15 cm to 8 cm.

Polyhydramnios is defined as an AFI of 25 cm or greater. Its cause is usually unknown, but it may be associated with fetal anomalies, insulin-dependent diabetes, gestational diabetes, or Rh isoimmunization. Fluid accumulation usually occurs slowly but it may also be acute, accruing in as little as 24 hours. It may interfere with maternal breathing. A clinical finding in cases of polyhydramnios is an inability to palpate the fetus. Preterm birth will occur in up to one third of the cases, but the underlying cause of polyhydramnios rather than excess fluid may determine whether or not PTL will occur (Many et al, 1995).

Biophysical Profile

A fourth test commonly used to evaluate fetal well-being is the BPP. This test uses ultrasound to assess the baby's muscle tone, movement, and breathing. The amount of amniotic fluid is evaluated also, using a criterion of at least one pocket of fluid measuring 2 cm in two perpendicular planes. A positive finding in each category is given a score of 2. Negative findings are given a score of 0. The four measurements are combined with results of the NST, 2 points being awarded when the nonstress test shows desired accelerations in the absence of worrisome decelerations. The desired score is 10/10. (Table 3-4.)

TABLE 3-4. Biophysical Profile Scoring: Technique and Interpretation*

Biophysical Variable	Normal Score	Abnormal (Score = 0)
Fetal breathing movements	At least 1 episode of FBM of at least 30-sec duration in 30-min observation	Absent FBM or no episode of ≥30 sec in 30 minutes
Gross body movement	At least 3 discrete body/limb movements in 30 min (episodes of active continuous movement considered as single movement)	2 or fewer episodes of body/limb movements in 30 min
Fetal tone	At least 1 episode of active extension with return to flexion of fetal limb(s) or trunk. Opening and closing of hand considered normal tone	Either slow extension with return to partial flexion or movement of limb in full extension or absent fetal movement with fetal hand held in complete or partial deflection
Reactive FHR	At least 2 episodes of FHR acceleration of ≥15 beat/min and of at least 15 sec-duration associated with fetal movement in 30 min	Less than 2 episodes of acceleration of FHR or acceleration of <15 beats/min in 30 min
Qualitative AFV†	At least 1 pocket of AF that measures at least 2 cm in 2 perpendicular planes	Either no AF pockets or a pocket <2 cm in two perpendicular planes

* FBM = fetal breathing movement; FHR = fetal heart rate; AFV = amniotic fluid volume; AF = amniotic fluid.

† Modification of the criteria for reduced amniotic fluid from <1 cm to <2 cm would seem reasonable.

From Manning, F. (1994). Fetal biophysical assessment by ultrasound. In R. Creasy and R.K. Resnik (Eds.), *Maternal-Fetal medicine: Principles and practice* (p. 345). Philadelphia: W.B. Saunders.

One or more of these tests for fetal well-being is also performed when

The expectant mother has a medical condition known to affect fetal outcome
The fetus is known to be at risk
A history of stillbirth is present
Labor does not occur within the expected time frame for term babies.

The appropriate time to initiate special studies in women who have had a stillborn baby has not been determined. In practice it is common to begin testing 2 to 3 weeks before the gestational age at which the stillbirth occurred. A recent recommendation based on a study of 300 patients suggests that antepartum surveillance be initiated at 32 weeks (Weeks et al, 1995).

Fetal well-being is also assessed as gestational age approaches 42 weeks, a time when the placenta may lose its ability to nourish the baby and fetal well-being may be jeopardized. These tests are usually initiated a few days before 42 weeks and may include an NST, an AFI, and a BPP. Because of data that con-

TABLE 3-5A. The Bishop Score

	0	1	2	3
Dilatation	0	1–2	3–4	5–6
Effacement	0–30	40–50	60–70	80
Station	−3	−2	−1	+1
Consistency of cervix	Firm	Medium	Soft	
Position	Posterior	Midline	Anterior	

clude that pregnancies carried beyond 42 weeks put babies at risk, labor is often induced at this time.

When an induction is anticipated, the cervix should be assessed to determine whether or not a cervical or vaginal medication might help "ripen" the cervix. Ripeness is determined by a vaginal examination to identify cervical dilatation and consistency, the position of the cervix in the vagina (anterior, mid, or posterior), effacement, and the station of the presenting part. This approach to cervical evaluation is called the "Bishop" score (Table 3-5). A score of 6 or more in a primigravida usually precludes the need for a ripening agent.

Do fetal well-being tests improve fetal outcome? The answer is unknown because too few randomized controlled trials have been conducted with samples large enough to detect benefits. There is wide variation in the behavior of the human fetus and the norms for evaluation are arbitrary. "How many movements, respirations, or accelerations? In what time period? . . . Abnormal results are seldom reliable, prompting most clinicians to use antenatal testing to forecast fetal *wellness* rather than *illness*" (Cunningham et al, 1993, p. 1041). Despite the shortcomings of antenatal testing, surveillance methods are widely used and are likely to be the standard of care in most communities.

TABLE 3-5B. Modified Bishop's Score

	Cm.	Score
Station	−3	0
	−2	1
	−1 or 0	2
	+1 or +2	3
Dilatation	0	0
	1–2	2
	3–4	4
	>4	6
Length of cervix	3	0
	2	1
	1	2
	0	3

Presentation

In the last trimester of pregnancy, the abdominal examination should identify the baby's presentation (the part of the fetus that lies over the pelvic inlet). Presentation may be cephalic (vertex), breech, face, or shoulder (Figure 3-7). Any presentation other than vertex at delivery increases the risk for poor perinatal outcome. Hopefully, any baby in a malpresentation will turn and be "head down" after the 37th week of pregnancy. If this has not occurred, refer the client to a clinician experienced in turning the baby to a vertex presentation. This procedure, called a *version*, should be done only with ultrasound monitoring of the fetal heart rate and availability of a Cesarean operation should fetal distress occur.

Clinicians are taught to use the four "Leopold's maneuvers" to identify not only the presentation of the baby, but also its position (the relationship of an arbitrarily chosen point on the presenting part to the right or left side of the maternal pelvis). Skilled clinicians are able, on some occasions, to gather the data intended by Leopold's maneuvers: the baby's presenting part and position, how much of the presenting part has descended into the pelvis, and whether or not the head is flexed.

Before labor, the most important information is identification of the presenting part at 37 weeks' gestation, a time at which an attempt can be made to convert the malpresentation to a vertex presentation. Obtain this information by grasping the uterine fundus between the thumb and middle finger of one hand. When something soft is felt, it is usually the buttocks; when something round, firm, and easily moved is felt, it is usually the fetal head. After determining which part of the baby is in the fundus, confirm your assessment by repeating the maneuver with the part of the baby that is in the pelvis.

Figure 3-8 describes the procedure for determining fetal presentation.

▶ HELPFUL HINT

> Babies are often in a posterior position prenatally. This has nothing to do with the position the baby will decide to use during labor, as most babies in a vertex presentation enter the pelvis in a transverse position regardless of the position they favored late in pregnancy. Because women who attend childbirth classes are often taught that posterior labors are long and difficult, hearing that her baby is in a posterior position late in pregnancy can cause the mother unnecessary worry. If the client asks about the baby's position, tell her the baby is in a perfect position or "just the right position" for this stage of pregnancy (unless, of course, the baby is breech or transverse).

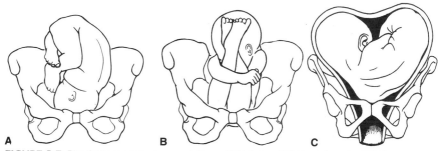

A **B** **C**

FIGURE 3-7. The fetus in various presentations. **(A)** Vertex. **(B)** Frank breech. **(C)** Transverse lie.

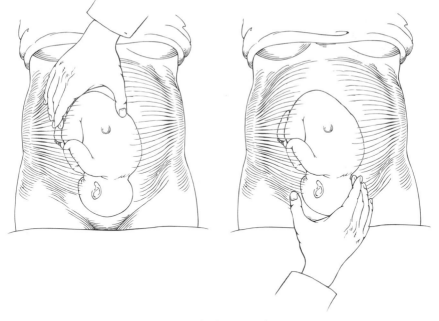

FIGURE 3-8. Procedure for determining fetal presentation.

Offer to draw a picture of the baby on your client's abdomen if she is at or greater than 32 weeks (or earlier). While those of us who do not consider ourselves artists may panic, anyone can do a drawing that a pregnant mother will like.

If you follow the lines as shown in Appendix R, you cannot go wrong. Practice on a piece of paper first. Follow the numbers unless you can do better on your own. Draw with a permanent marker (a "Sharpie" laundry marker works well and dries in a few seconds). As you become proficient, try drawing 5 fingers and toes, an ear, and hair. The drawing will last up to 3 days. Most women will be delighted with your artwork; some will have someone take a picture of their belly, and put the picture in the baby book. (Appendix R also contains realistic figures, drawn by Polly Malby, CNM.) You may wish to keep the drawings taped to a wall in the examining room to use as a guide. For many, this visual image helps to make the baby real, and some women report that the drawing facilitated attachment to the baby.

Of course, some women will not want you to draw on their abdomen and their wishes should be respected. However, most women appreciate at least one drawing, and some want it done at each visit.

▼ Laboratory Tests

Maternal Serum Multiple Marker Screening

Alphafetoprotein is a glycoprotein synthesized by the fetus and excreted by the fetal liver. When the neural tube fails to close in the early days after conception, nonintact fetal skin allows the protein to leak from fetal capillaries into the amniotic fluid, where it crosses fetal membranes and enters the maternal circulation. Maternal blood levels of alphafetoprotein then become elevated. Anencephaly, encephalocele, and spina bifida are the most frequently neural tube defects; they occur within 28 days of conception.

While alphafetoprotein testing was used initially to screen only for neural tube defects, continued research demonstrated that low levels can predict up to one fourth of Down syndrome cases in women under 35 at the time of delivery. When unconjugated estriol and chorionic gonadotropin are measured at the same time MSAFP levels are determined, sensitivity in identifying Down syndrome is increased to approximately 60% (Busch & Himes, 1995). The level of MSAFP in maternal blood is expressed as "multiples of the median" (MOM). Levels of 2.5 MOM or greater indicate increased risk for open neural tube defects. MSAFP testing can identify 90% of anencephaly and up to 85% of spina bifida. The concentration of chorionic gonadotropin, a placental hormone, is nearly twice as high when Down syndrome is present. Maternal serum concentration of unconjugated estriol is about 25% lower.

When MSAFP, unconjugated estriol, and chorionic gonadotropin are all measured, this test is commonly known as maternal serum multiple marker screening, the triple test, AFP plus, marker test, triple screen, or prenatal risk profile. When levels are high enough to suspect a neural tube defect, or low enough to wonder about Down syndrome, amniocentesis can be performed.

Reliable test results depend on an accurate assessment of gestational age and maternal weight, as MSAFP values normally increase as pregnancy progresses, and a dilutional effect resulting in an incorrectly low value could occur in heavy women. Abnormal values will be obtained if gestational age is inaccurate or if more than one fetus is present. Accordingly, before amniocentesis is performed, an abnormal multiple marker screen should be followed by an ultrasound examination for gestational age and structural abnormalities, if one has not been performed previously.

The test should be performed between 15 and 18 weeks' gestation, although some laboratories are able to test through the 20th week. Because the test is only a screening test, false-positive results will occur. Women who have not had an ultrasound before the test is performed should know that most of the positive tests are the result of inaccurate dating. Most women with positive results have normal, healthy babies. All women need to know that the test does not detect all cases of Down syndrome. Nor does it detect most other types of anomalies.

Recently, an association between trisomy 18 and lowered levels of all three analytes in the multiple marker screen has been noted. Trisomy 18 is a severe chromosomal abnormality that occurs approximately once in 8000 live births. Figure 3-9 outlines the activities appropriate when performing the maternal serum multiple marker test.

When an abnormal test is reported, it is very important to tell a woman more than "The test is abnormal. You need to go for genetic counseling." Interpret the risks in the way that will be best understood by the client. A helpful approach may be to translate the numbers into a percentage that reflects the chances for a healthy baby. For example, if a woman's chances of having a baby with Down syndrome are 1 in 267, she has a 99.5% chance of having a normal baby. A 1 in 50 chance of having a baby with a chromosomal abnormality is still a 98% chance of having a healthy baby.

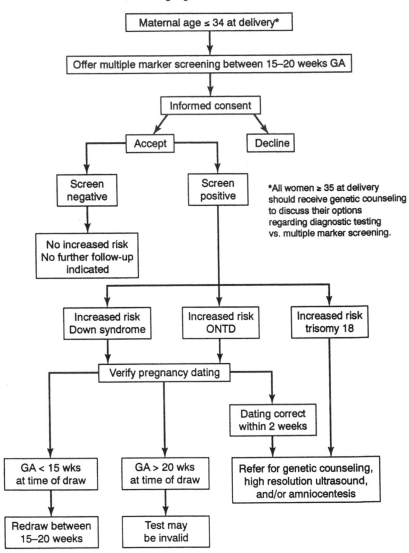

FIGURE 3-9. Algorithm for multiple marker screening.

Glucose Screening

In many practices throughout the United States, all pregnant women are screened for gestational diabetes at 26 to 28 weeks' gestation. The client drinks a liquid containing 50 g of glucose. Women with an abnormal value undergo further testing with a 100-g glucose tolerance test. Abnormal values on this test are used to diagnose gestational diabetes mellitus (GDM).

Those who believe in screening all pregnant women for gestational diabetes believe that macrosomia can be prevented by administering insulin to the approximately 10% of pregnant women diagnosed as gestational diabetics who have persistently high fasting glucose levels despite following a diabetic diet. Macrosomia poses problems for both mother and baby. Mothers have an increased chance of Cesarean birth or, if the birth is vaginal, an increased chance of trauma to maternal tissue. Macrosomic babies are more likely to have birth trauma and hypoglycemia.

While universal screening for GDM is "standard of care" in many communities, the practice may be questioned because, on retesting, 50% to 70% of women with two or more abnormal values on the 100-g test will have normal values (Enkin et al, 1995, p. 58). In addition, most macrosomic babies are born to women who were overweight at the start of pregnancy, have excessive weight gains during pregnancy, or are post-dates (Enkin et al, 1995, p. 58), rather than to women diagnosed as having gestational diabetes.

The Screening Test for Gestational Diabetes

Fasting before the 50-g screening test is not required. Thresholds commonly used to identify women requiring further testing vary by institution. They include glucose levels of 130 mg/dL; 135 mg/dL; and 140 mg/dL. When the chosen threshold is reached, a 3-hour test, the glucose tolerance test, is ordered.

The Diagnostic Test

The diagnostic test for GDM is administered after a fast of at least 8 hours. For 3 days prior to the test, a high-carbohydrate diet should be ingested. At least 150 g per day of carbohydrate is recommended, as the insulin of women on carbohydrate-restricted diets may be slower to respond to the glucose and an abnormal result is more likely. An easy way for some women to eat sufficient carbohydrates is to consume 4 extra slices of bread for each of the 3 days. On the day of the test, water may be consumed, but cigarettes should be avoided.

The client is given 100 g of glucose orally in the same kind of drink used in the 1-hour test. Norms commonly accepted for the 3-hour test are shown in Box 3-7. Gestational diabetes is diagnosed when two or more values are met or exceeded. If a woman vomits after ingesting this much glucose, do not ask her to repeat the test. Instead, follow her fasting glucose levels at each prenatal visit. Do not use random glucose testing, as it provides no pertinent information.

The management of women with GDM varies greatly. In some places women are placed on a diabetic diet and have a fasting blood sugar performed only at regular clinic visits. As long as the fasting blood sugar is below 105 mg/dL, no other testing is performed until 40 weeks, when tests of fetal well-being are initiated. (Nonstress tests are usually scheduled biweekly starting at 40 weeks' gestation for women with GDM, as the placentas of these women may deteriorate prematurely.) Persistent fasting blood glucose levels of

Box 3-7. Norms for the 3-Hour Glucose Tolerance Test for the Diagnosis of Gestational Diabetes*' **	
Fasting	105 mg/dL***
1 hour	190 mg/dL
2 hours	165 mg/dL
3 hours	145 mg/dL

* Two abnormal values are necessary for a diagnosis.
** Some practices will use other values, especially for the fasting level.
*** Some practices use a fasting blood sugar of 90 or 95 mg/dL rather than 105 mg/dL.

105 mg/dL or above, after 2 weeks of a diabetic diet, identify the women who usually will be given insulin.

In some practices women are not only placed on a diabetic diet but are asked to monitor their blood glucose at home as often as 4 times a day. Their clinic visit is supplemented with a 2-hour postprandial test in addition to a fasting blood sugar. Norms for the 2-hour postprandial test vary between 120 mg/dL and 140 mg/dL.

Some practitioners feel that women with very high blood glucose levels with the 50-g screening test should not have the 3-hour test because their chance of having GDM probably approaches 95%. Levels above 182 mg/dL fall into this category. Other practitioners feel that a diagnosis is necessary so that women without GDM do not unnecessarily have to follow the diet, have extra blood tests performed, and undergo NST or induction.

Women who enter care already overweight (20% greater than ideal weight for height) are more likely to have problems metabolizing glucose in pregnancy. Therefore, if you believe in screening for GDM, request a 1-hour screening glucose test at the initial prenatal visit of overweight women, and repeat the test in the last trimester.

Urine Testing for Protein and Glucose With Reagent Strips

Proteinuria

Reagent strips are routinely used to test a random sample of urine for protein at each prenatal visit to screen for preeclampsia and UTI. Color changes distinguish between varying amounts of protein (1+ = 30 mg; 2+ = 100 mg; 3+ = 300 mg; and 4+ = >2000 mg). Unfortunately, both false-positive and false-negative results are common with reagent strip testing. In a retrospective chart review of pregnant women hospitalized for high BP, "Dipstick protein values of 1+ were associated with a wide range of quantitative protein excretion from 94.2 to 8100 mg in a 24-hour collection." Additionally, when reagent strip values were ≥2+, there was a 10.5% false-positive rate (Meyer et al, 1994). The imprecision of urine reagent strips for detecting the amount of protein in the urine is partly because assigning a value is based on subtle color changes, and partly because protein excretion varies throughout the day.

While the U.S. Public Health Service report on the content of prenatal care could find no evidence to support routine urine testing with reagent strips (U.S. Public Health Service, 1989), the practice continues in most prenatal care settings. To maximize the test's accuracy, obtain a clean-catch specimen when a random urine specimen contains a trace or more protein because the sample may have been contaminated with vaginal discharge or blood. It can be helpful to gently insert a vaginal tampon before cleansing the vulva to ensure a more valid specimen. This may be particularly useful with obese women who find it hard to reach their vulva for appropriate cleaning. Do not ask the client to drink water so that she can void sooner, as this will dilute the specimen and can give a false-negative result. While trace amounts of protein in a urine specimen are often considered insignificant, remember that both negative and trace results in women with high BP may miss women with significant proteinuria.

Although proteinuria of ≥5 gm per day is virtually excluded by the presence of negative or trace protein on dipstick, negative or trace values were found in 81 of 243 pregnancies with mild proteinuria (sensitivity of dipstick ≥1+ equals 67%) and should not be used to rule out significant proteinuria . . . (Meyer et al, 1994, p. 139).

Unfortunately, the authors of the above study did not state whether or not the urine samples tested with reagent strips were random-voided or clean-catch specimens.

If the clean-catch urine specimen tests positive, inquire about symptoms of a UTI and preeclampsia. Look for a BP elevation, rapid weight gain, and edema. Use a reagent strip, if possible, to test for a UTI, as proteinuria may be due to bacteria in the urine. Consider kidney disease if proteinuria is the only finding.

▶ SOMETHING FUN

Teach pregnant women to test their own urine with the reagent test strip and note the results in their record.

Glucosuria

The same reagent strip used to test urine for protein usually contains a second reagent that tests for glucose. A clean-catch specimen of urine is not required for accurate results. Be careful about assuming that glucosuria in a pregnant woman can be attributed to a recent diet high in sugar. Because glucosuria in the first two trimesters is associated with a higher incidence of gestational diabetes, providers who believe GDM can affect the outcome of pregnancy should request a 1-hour glucose screen as soon as glucosuria is identified. Third trimester glucosuria found after a normal 1-hour glucose screen at 24 to 28 weeks' gestation has not been found to be significant, and no additional testing is indicated (Gribble et al, 1995).

Screening for Group B Streptococcus (GBS)

Some practices have routinely obtained vaginal cultures at 26 to 28 weeks' gestation to screen for group B streptococcus (GBS) infection. Neonatal sepsis caused by *Streptococcus agalactiae*, Group B streptococcus, is a common cause of severe morbidity and mortality in newborns. Because of the devastating nature of this illness and the effectiveness of intrapartum, IV antibiotics in preventing its transmission to the newborn, the American Academy of Pediatrics (AAP) has recommended that all pregnant women be screened for GBS at 26 to 28 weeks' gestation with a culture of the lower vagina and anorectum.

Women who test positive prenatally and who have additional risk factors (premature rupture of membranes before 37 weeks, PTL, fever during labor, multiple gestation, rupture of membranes for more than 18 hours) are to be treated with antibiotics during labor (Committee on Infectious Diseases and Committee on Fetus and Newborn, 1992). This policy is a subject of discussion and controversy because it causes many women to receive antibiotics in labor, although only 1% to 2% of infants who are colonized develop sepsis, pneumonia, or meningitis.

Colonization rates for GBS vary across the United States, from 3% to 4% in some Latina populations, to 40% in populations with high rates of STDs. Two thirds of women who are culture-positive prenatally will be culture-negative at delivery without treatment, and up to 13% of the women who have negative cultures prenatally will be positive at delivery (Agnoli, 1994). Administering oral antibiotics prenatally eradicates GBS, but only temporarily. There is a high spontaneous recolonization rate after antibiotics are discontinued.

Guidelines published by the CDC in 1996 recommended one of two approaches to perinatal Group B streptococcal disease:

A screening-based approach (Figure 3-10), a strategy that screens all pregnant women late in the third trimester as a basis for deciding on antibiotics in labor

A risk-factor approach, a strategy that uses intrapartum risk factors alone as a basis for decision-making in regard to the use of antibiotics in labor (CDC, 1996b).

Remember that the specimen for the group B strep culture should be obtained from the lower (outer) third of the vagina and from the perianal/anal area. Insertion of a speculum is not necessary to obtain the vaginal specimen.

▼ Health Education

An essential part of health education at the prenatal revisit is determining whether or not the client is aware of essential information. For instance, does she know the danger signs for her trimester of pregnancy, whom to contact in an emergency, and important phone numbers? Depending on gestational age, does she know the two "magic numbers": 6 contractions per hour (appropriate to discuss after 20 weeks) and the number of fetal movements per time period your practice has selected as the "movement alarm signal" (appropriate to discuss after 24 weeks).

Many topics are appropriate to discuss at return prenatal visits. A helpful way to choose subjects is to offer the client a list from which to choose. Topics can be checked off when they are covered.

Planning for Labor and Birth

A traditional component of midwifery practice has always involved helping women and their families prepare for labor and birth. Thoughts about how this should be done vary. For some, preparation continues to be through childbirth education classes.

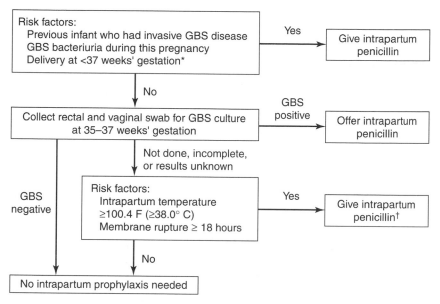

* If membranes ruptured at <37 weeks' gestation, and the mother has not begun labor, collect group B streptococcal culture and either a) administer antibiotics until cultures are completed and the results are negative or b) begin antibiotics only when positive cultures are available. No prophylaxis is needed if culture obtained at 35–37 weeks' gestation was negative.

† Broader spectrum antibiotics may be considered at the physician's discretion, based on clinical indications.

FIGURE 3-10. *Algorithm for prevention of early-onset of Group B streptococcus disease (GBS) in neonates, using prenatal screening at 35–37 weeks gestation. From CDC. (1996). Prevention of perinatal group B streptococcal disease: A public health perspective.* Morbidity and Mortality Weekly Report, 45(RR-7), 1–24.

Childbirth Education

Obstetrics care changed in this country in the 1960s, when expectant mothers organized for the first time, using their collective will to have a voice in the way they were allowed to labor and give birth. Before this, almost all women in the United States received an amnesic drug and heavy doses of narcotics when they went into labor. The reversal of this approach to pain relief in labor began in the 1940s when an English physician, Grantley Dick-Read, wrote *Childbirth Without Fear*. This book was read by relatively few women, but it was the first of a number of books including *Thank You, Dr. Lamaze* by Marjorie Karmel, and *Six Practical Lessons to an Easier Childbirth* by Elisabeth Bing. Taken together, these books provided hope and encouragement to increasing numbers of women who wanted to be actively involved in the birth process. This approach came to be known as natural childbirth. It emphasized group classes to provide class participants with information about the process of labor, and guided practice in breathing techniques that were thought to decrease pain.

While most physicians initially disliked these classes, and some refused to sign the permission slip that women often needed to participate in them, over time childbirth education classes became the "ticket" that permitted a husband to be at his wife's side when she labored and gave birth. Today, classes are available emphasizing these same aspects. However, other classes that use a more eclectic and/or individualized approach are available in many communities.

The role of the health care provider is to work with each pregnant woman to help her determine what she feels is most appropriate for her. Questions such as "What is important for you when you are in labor and giving birth? Have you thought about how you would like it to go, how you think it will go? Have you thought about how you would like to welcome your baby?" can stimulate the mother's thinking.

When it appears that childbirth education classes might be helpful, share your knowledge about community resources. This information is best obtained from talking with childbirth educators about their philosophy and teaching approach. Other helpful information includes the cost, location, and timing of classes. Some communities offer classes both day and evening, including sunrise classes for those who find it best to attend class before work or school. Weekend classes, often offered at a resort, allow parents-to-be to have a concentrated period of time to think about labor and birth. Some classes emphasize patterned breathing. Some use techniques of hypnosis or visualization. Others stress "finding your own way through labor" and present a variety of tools that may be helpful. The more the clinician knows about the various classes offered in the community, the easier and more likely it will be that the client will find a group that fits her interests, personality, and learning style.

Women who choose not to attend classes and women who are unable to participate in a formal series may appreciate help with breathing techniques at their prenatal visits. You might begin with something like this for women who express an interest in visualization.

Think of labor as you would an athletic event. It will help if you relax, pace yourself, conserve energy. Remember to keep breathing. Notice those things that help you relax and feel confident. Think of your cervix and vagina as being soft and stretchy in front of the baby. Imagine the baby coming down against soft, stretchy tissues. Think of yourself as healthy and strong and capable. Take one contraction at a time and one event, one change at a time. Help will be available when you need it. (From Virginia Capan, CNM, personal communication.)

Any discussion about pain relief in labor must consider the clinician's own attitudes and biases about the nature and purpose of labor and the potential value of birthing without medicine to relieve pain. Inevitably, these personal beliefs influence recommendations to the client. When the person providing prenatal care will not be the client's birth attendant, the attitudes and practices of those likely to be assisting at the birth should be known and communicated to clients.

Pain medication in labor should also be discussed among all providers who, as a group, attend births. Questions for discussion might include:

What special needs in regard to pain relief in labor might exist for women whose lives have always been characterized by pain—poor women, for example, or women who have been abused?

When is it appropriate to deny pain medication to women in labor who ask for it?

Are a certain group of women giving birth in hospital settings perceived as not needing pain medication in labor?

Should women be offered pain relief medication if they do not ask for it?

Some women are certain from the start that they want an epidural anesthetic early in labor. Some women are committed to doing without any kind of pharmacologic assistance. Some women want to keep their options open. The provider, then, must work with the client to determine the most appropriate way to get ready for labor and birth.

Clinicians may be uncertain about when to encourage women to consider a birth without analgesia or anesthesia, and when to know that it truly is in a woman's best interests to support her decision to use pharmacologic relief measures. The provider must remember that preparation for labor takes place within the client herself. "Fight or flight," the hormones of fear and guardedness, counteract labor and inhibit the progress of dilatation. Perhaps one of the most important contributions the provider can make is to act to help the client be confident in her own decisions.

Midwives come from a long tradition of helping women labor without pain medicine. Many have personally experienced the power and satisfaction that have come from that experience. But the women served in hospitals today have personal needs that are not always best served by minimal amounts or no analgesia. Clinicians must acknowledge these needs and individual differences in their clients. Among other things, be aware that

> . . . working-class and middle-class woman have different attitudes toward childbirth during pregnancy, different experiences during childbirth, and different post-partum evaluations of their childbirth experiences. A single set of prescriptions for childbirth may not, therefore, be appropriate for all women (Nelson, 1983, p. 284).

The Birth Plan

It is common practice in some places to ask the expectant mother to put her desires for labor and birth in writing. This document is called a birth plan. (See Appendix S for a sample.) Some birth plan forms are brief while others are long and detailed. Some health care providers find them helpful, and others wish they had never been invented. Whether or not a written birth plan is encouraged, take time to help the client consider whom she wants with her during labor and at the birth, and how she thinks she will react to the practices and procedures she is likely to encounter. Suggest that she choose people with whom she can be comfortable, and whom she trusts with sounds, pain, body exposure, and intimacy.

When possible, request a meeting between you, the client, and all the people she hopes will be present during labor or at the birth. Reviewing the expectant mother's desires out loud and hearing each person's questions, expectations, hopes, and fears can clear the air and set the stage for a supportive birth experience. The health care provider may want to review the process of labor with the group, emphasizing how different it is for each person. Talk about long labors and short labors, membranes rupturing before contractions begin and membranes rupturing just before the birth. Allow those who have given or witnessed birth to express some of their thoughts. End by asking the expectant mother if there is anything about her that those who attend the birth should know or would find helpful.

Some birth attendants feel that everyone present during labor should be "doing" something "useful." Birth attendants may also want partners to become "coaches" during labor. This role may or may not be appropriate. A small, ex-

ploratory study has shown that some men readily assume the role of coach or
teammate. More, however, are likely to be "witnesses" or "companions." Health
care providers can enhance the birth experience by explaining that all roles are
legitimate to assume and that the roles assumed should be compatible with the
personalities, hopes, and relationships of those involved with the patient
(Chapman, 1992). Hopefully, all birth attendants will remember that the birth
belongs to the laboring woman. "Doing" is not always the best thing to "do."
Sometimes merely "being" is a very useful—and therapeutic—activity. Above
all, the clinician should aim at giving a woman as much control as possible in
what is a complex, dynamic, painful process.

Preparing Other Children

The arrival of a new baby will have a profound effect on every member of the
family. Parents with other children often appreciate help in two areas: explaining how the baby got into mom's uterus, and preparing a child for the arrival of
a new sister or brother.

Appendix T contains two guides for parents: "How Does the Baby Get Out?
(And How Did He get in There Anyway?)" and "Helping Your Child Become a
Big Sister or Brother." (These documents were written by Marie Brown, CNM,
Portland, OR and may be reproduced if no charge is imposed and appropriate
credit is given to the author.)

Honoring the Expectant Mother

Clinicians play an important role in helping pregnant women feel special. For example, you might bring special cups for your practice setting. Offer women tea or
juice when they come for a prenatal visit. Sit for a minute and enjoy a cup yourself. When time permits, offer your client a back rub or a foot massage. Wear
something unique—a hat, an appropriate t-shirt. Have a tray of fruit available.

In some situations, you may wish to suggest a special ceremony to honor the
expectant mother and provide her with emotional support. This ceremony is
one that she can plan with you, by herself, or one that she can ask friends or family to offer for her. A "blessing way," a ceremony similar to that celebrated by
some pregnant Native American women, may be helpful.

A blessing ceremony is usually attended by close female friends of the expectant mother, although male partners and friends can also be invited. One
version has participants offer gifts designed to remind the woman when she is
in labor that her friends are thinking of her and sharing their strength and wisdom. Each participant may bring an item to put on a necklace that the woman
will wear while she labors, or small objects to put into a wreath that the mother
will take to the place of birth. The participants might gather in a circle united
with the expectant mother by a cord (often made of yarn or string) that is passed
around a wrist of each person. The participants may tell the mother-to-be what
they admire most about her, what they wish for her, and which of their own
strengths they will be wishing for her while she is in labor. Each then breaks the
cord at her wrist and wears the cord until the baby is born. Often the blessing
way ends with the establishment of a telephone tree so that everyone present at
the blessing way can be contacted when the honoree's labor begins. Each participant can then focus intently on the mother in the hours ahead.

It is fun to develop personal variations on this theme. If the expectant mother
likes flowers and gardening, the participants can bring her a plant or a basket of
hyacinth or freesia bulbs in a shallow pan of water. Start the bulbs at a time

when they will flower a few days after the due date. If the mother has not yet given birth, the flowers may cheer her when the last days seem endless.

Client Teaching

Teaching should be an integral component of prenatal care. Pamphlets, booklets, and brochures are often given to clients to take the place of or supplement teaching by the health care provider. Visual aids may also be used to facilitate client learning. Key points in providing this information include:

- Introducing topics at appropriate times
- Being aware of the client's literacy level
- Using audiovisual aids to increase understanding by clients who are visual learners
- Realizing that giving information cannot always be equated with learning.

Audiovisual Aids

Audio and visual aids are available from a variety of sources. Many libraries have extensive collections of books on birth and parenting. Some lend videotapes depicting labor and birth. Helpful visual aids for the clinic or office setting include the following:

Fetal models that represent the size of the fetus at 10, 12, 15, and 20 weeks: While generally accurate in regard to size, these models have facial features that are more distinct than actual features at these gestational ages. Still, the models are useful. (about $20 each)

A cloth model of the pelvis: This model allows pregnant women to visualize their pelvis and one of the holes through which the baby must travel during labor. The cream-colored cloth of the model is "splotched" with brown to suggest anatomical landmarks. Women with low literacy skills may find the splotches confusing. (about $55)

A knitted uterus and vagina: This model can demonstrate how the cervix effaces and dilates and how the baby passes through the vagina. When a doll is placed inside the uterus, the procedure for "stripping membranes" can also be demonstrated. A Cesarean version is available. Directions for knitting the uterus and vagina are also available. The advantage to knitting your own uterus is that you can select an appropriate color of yarn. Most of the knitted models come in stripes or the color blue. ($21; $23 for Cesarean version; $2 for knitting directions)

Models of the placenta, cord, and membranes: These models can help clients understand how the baby fits in the amniotic fluid sac and is surrounded by amniotic fluid. They also can be used to explain what the placenta looks like, how it is attached to the uterus, how the cord is clamped, and how the placenta separates. The fetal model, the size of a full-term baby, has an umbilical cord that snaps on to the umbilicus at one end and to a placenta at the other end. The baby fits inside a gauze sac that closes with a drawstring. These models are also available in a 7-inch size that can fit inside a large pocket. (about $43; about $48 for the 7-inch model)

A flat model of a full-term baby made out of plastic: This jointed model allows the head and extremities to move. It can be placed on the mother's abdomen during prenatal visits in the last trimester to illustrate fetal position. The model also facilitates drawing a picture of the baby on the mother's abdomen for those who are reluctant to try the drawing on their own. (about $20)

All of the above are available from Childbirth Graphics, 1-800-299-3366, extension 287; fax: 817-751-0221.

A T-shirt with a model of a full-term baby in the uterus: This T-shirt can serve to illustrate that, toward the end of pregnancy, the baby usually lives head-down in the uterus. It is helpful to women and families who find it difficult to visualize the baby in the uterus. In institutions where clinic sessions are informal, it is fun to wear this T-shirt once in a while. It is available for about $10 from International Childbirth Education Association, 1-800-624-4934; fax: 612-854-8772.

Clients Who Can't Read

Most health care professionals assume that the majority of their clients are functionally literate (ie, able to read, write, and perform arithmetic computations at a level that permits them to use them in everyday life). However, in a study conducted in two urban public hospitals, as many as three fifths of the clients were found to have inadequate or marginal literacy in regard to their ability to use the health system to their advantage (Williams et al, 1995).

Level of education is sometimes used to estimate a person's literacy level. Generally speaking, adults with less education are less able to understand and use printed information than adults with more education (Kirsch et al, 1993). In the United States, 1 person in 5 reads at the 5th grade level or below. Among inner-city minorities, almost 2 out of 5 read below the 5th grade level. This is important to remember because

> Poor readers obtain much less from health care instructions than do skilled readers. This is true even for materials that have fairly low readability levels. Poor readers may read most or all of the words in an instruction and still obtain little or no meaning from the text (Doak et al, 1996).

Most health education material is written by good readers for good readers. An evaluation of client education pamphlets published by the American College of Obstetricians and Gynecologists found that 61 out of 74 pamphlets had a reading difficulty level of 11th grade or higher at a time when the mean literacy level was at or below the 8th grade (Zion & Aiman, 1989). Health care providers, then, must be aware not only of the client's literacy level, but of the reading level of any written material offered. In addition, since research has shown that women with low literacy skills have difficulty with particular words (Appendix U), clinicians should carefully choose the words they use.

People who find reading difficult frequently are embarrassed because they cannot read. They often go to great lengths to hide this problem and clinicians, as a result, find it difficult to identify clients with inadequate or marginal literacy skills. While literacy evaluation tests have been used in research studies to identify literacy level, no one test currently available is easily adaptable and sufficiently comprehensive to be useful in clinic and office settings. Consequently, clinicians are left to their own devices as they attempt to make good decisions about how to identify the client's literacy level and how to teach clients whose skills are low. Pamphlets and brochures, perhaps the most common vehicles for client teaching, may be inappropriate. The following guidelines may be helpful.

- Be aware that low literacy level is a silent but common problem.
- Make no assumptions about who can read and who cannot.
- Experiment with different ways of determining literacy level. You might try saying "Some people find it hard to understand what they read. Is this true for you?" or ask "Do you like to read?" or "Do you read very much?" Most illiterate women will say "No." (Be careful, however, not to assume that women who say "no" are illiterate.)
- Personally evaluate any brochures, pamphlets, and other materials that you give to clients, even when they have been specifically designed for women who cannot read well. An excellent book to guide evaluations of health education materials is *Teaching Patients with Low Literacy Skills* (Doak et al, 1996). Appendix V, taken from the book, lists points to consider when evaluating printed health education material for clients.
- Poor readers may understand and remember better with visual aids.
- Avoid using direct translations when using material that has been translated from another language. It is not possible to translate a document word-for-word and have the meaning be the same in both languages (Doak et al, 1996, p. 67; Fullerton et al, 1993).
- Establish whether or not a client understands your directions by asking her to restate your instructions. Giving information does not guarantee comprehension.

Clinicians also would do well to address learning style when teaching clients. People learn best when the teaching approach fits their learning style. The spoken word helps auditory learners, visual aids help visual learners, and manipulating materials helps kinesthetic learners. Many clients find combinations of these approaches helpful.

See Appendix W for sample client education materials. They may be reproduced if appropriate credit is given and no charge is made to the client.

▼ Conclusion

Good prenatal care requires a combination of knowledge, manual dexterity, respect for both the normal and the abnormal, good judgment, resourcefulness, compassion, and an appreciation of the lives of women. Thoughtful consideration of the uniqueness of each pregnant woman can lead to the provision of meaningful and useful health education.

4

The Postpartum Period

Immediately after birth profound changes take place in the mother's body and, frequently, in her heart, soul, and mind, as well. While health care providers may assume that the difficult part, labor, is over, many women find that it is just beginning.

The postpartum checkup is usually scheduled 6 weeks after birth, but with an awareness of the many issues that arise following the birth of a baby, earlier contact between the client and the health care provider is generally recommended.

▼ Postpartum Morbidity

Infection

Morbidity in the first postpartum weeks is usually due to endometritis, mastitis, or an infection of an episiotomy or laceration. Urinary tract infections (UTIs) and other illnesses, including pneumonia and influenza, can also occur and must be considered as well. In most instances, any postpartum woman who complains of fever with or without pain should be evaluated with a head to toe examination. Send a urine specimen for culture to rule out pyelonephritis. Cervical or vaginal cultures are not obtained routinely. Although a complete blood count (CBC) may be ordered, results are not easy to interpret if the infection occurs in the early postpartum days, since leucocyte counts are normally high at this time.

The decision to treat a woman with a postpartum infection as an outpatient should be made on the basis of how sick she appears. What is her temperature? Her pulse? The leucocyte count? Is there an adult at home who can look after her while she is ill?

Endometritis

A woman with endometritis usually presents with fever, abdominal pain, and foul-smelling lochia. Examination of the abdomen will reveal a tender uterus. Consult with a physician when endometritis occurs. Hospitalization for intravenous (IV) antibiotics may be necessary if the client presents with a high fever and rapid pulse. Outpatient treatment is summarized in Box 4-1.

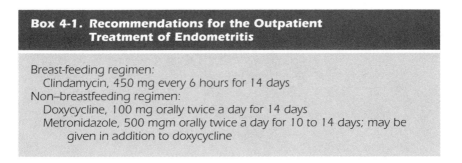

Box 4-1. Recommendations for the Outpatient Treatment of Endometritis

Breast-feeding regimen:
    Clindamycin, 450 mg every 6 hours for 14 days
Non–breastfeeding regimen:
    Doxycycline, 100 mg orally twice a day for 14 days
    Metronidazole, 500 mgm orally twice a day for 10 to 14 days; may be
        given in addition to doxycycline

Mastitis

Mastitis can occur any time when a woman is breastfeeding, but it usually does not occur before the 10th postpartum day. The causative organism is usually *Staphylococcus aureus*, and new mothers commonly confuse symptoms with those of flu. Your client is likely to tell you she aches all over and feels like she has been "hit by a truck." She typically has a fever of 101°F or more.

Treatment of mastitis is summarized in Box 4-2. Women with mastitis should feel significantly better within 24 hours of taking antibiotics. If they do not, they may need to be hospitalized for IV antibiotics.

Comfort measures include bedrest for at least 24 hours, moist heat to the infected breast for 20 to 30 minutes every 2 to 3 hours while awake, and acetaminophen for pain and fever. The mother should drink plenty of liquids and discontinue use of a bra for a few days, unless she experiences discomfort without one. A bra, particularly one with an underwire, may increase discomfort.

Mastitis does not contaminate the mother's milk. The baby should continue to nurse from both breasts. In fact, frequent nursing decreases the chances that a breast abscess will form. Feeding from the unaffected breast first usually is helpful. If feeding from the affected breast is too painful, a breast pump or manual expression of the milk is often necessary to prevent engorgement and continue milk production.

Wound Infection

An infected laceration or episiotomy will appear red and swollen. Purulent discharge will be present. The repair may have "broken down." Often sitz baths 3 to 4 times a day and a local antibiotic cream to the infected skin area are all that is needed. In other instances, the wound should be opened by removing the stitches and then cleansed with normal saline. Oral antibiotics such as clindamycin should be administered. Note skin color around the episiotomy site, as necrosis can occur.

Urinary Tract Infection

A UTI also may be a source of postpartum morbidity, and should be considered in a differential diagnosis of postpartum fever or pain and aching.

When antibiotics are given postpartally, a new mother may develop a yeast infection of the nipples. Presenting symptoms are bilateral nipple pain or sensitivity, rosy pink nipples, pins-and-needles pain in the breasts, and, sometimes,

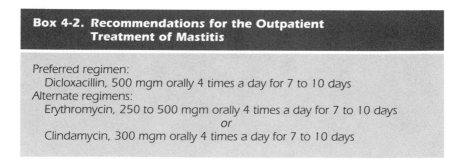

Box 4-2. Recommendations for the Outpatient Treatment of Mastitis

Preferred regimen:
  Dicloxacillin, 500 mgm orally 4 times a day for 7 to 10 days
Alternate regimens:
  Erythromycin, 250 to 500 mgm orally 4 times a day for 7 to 10 days
            or
  Clindamycin, 300 mgm orally 4 times a day for 7 to 10 days

peeling skin on the nipples. The baby may have oral thrush and a bright red monilia diaper rash. Advise the mother to apply Nystatin cream to the nipples (3 times a day for 7 days) and wash all pacifiers and parts of a breast pump with hot water. The baby can be given 1 cc of Nystatin suspension orally 4 times a day for 14 days. Do not recommend that the mother apply the baby's Nystatin to her nipples. The suspension is sticky when it dries, and the mother's bra will stick to it. Treat mother's nipples, baby's mouth, and baby's bottom until all three are clear for 48 hours.

Because there may be drug resistance to Nystatin, Lotrimin cream applied twice a day may be the drug of choice in some communities for both mother's nipples and baby's bottom. When Lotrimin cream is used, the baby will still need oral Nystatin. Gentian violet is messy but also appropriate.

Before prescribing any medication for women who are breastfeeding, be certain that the medication is safe. A helpful guide is *Medicine and Mothers Milk* (T. Hale, 1994, Amarillo, TX: Pharmasoft Medical Publications). This book can be ordered for about $20 from the publisher at 4606 Oregon, Amarillo, TX, 79107, 1-800-378-1317.

▼ Breast Problems

Engorgement

At times it is difficult to differentiate between mastitis, engorgement, and a plugged milk duct. Engorgement is usually bilateral, comes on gradually, causes a low-grade fever, and is not associated with any systemic symptoms. The breasts are usually warm to the touch and have a shiny appearance. Except for breast discomfort, mothers generally feel well unless the engorgement is severe, includes the breast's tail of Spence, and extends into the axilla. When the engorgement is this severe, mothers have to hold their arms away from the body to avoid pressure on the swollen breast tissue.

Treatment for engorgement in a breastfeeding mother is a mild analgesic, moist heat, and frequent nursing. Unfortunately, the swollen breast often makes it difficult for the baby to latch on to the nipple. In these cases, manual expression of milk or a breast pump to remove enough milk to soften the areola can help the baby nurse. Standing under a warm shower while manually expressing or pumping can also be helpful. There are many kinds of hand-held breast pumps available. Unfortunately, the least expensive also may work least well. *The Breastfeeding Triage Tool*, by Sandra Jolley (available for about $12 from Breastfeeding Publications, Seattle–King County Department of Public Health, 110 Prefontaine Ave. South, Suite 500, Seattle, WA, 98104) is a small, helpful, reference book about breastfeeding problems. The author discusses the causes of common problems, details how to assess and cope with these situations, and evaluates various kinds of breast pumps.

Engorgement in a bottlefeeding mother can be treated with analgesics and ice.

Plugged Duct

A plugged duct can also cause breast pain. The pain is usually confined to one breast and little or no warmth is present. If fever is present, it is low-grade. Mothers feel well. Heat packs, gentle massage of the breast toward the nipple, and varying positions for nursing the baby, help.

Nipple Pain

Nipple pain is common in breastfeeding women. In one study, 96 out of 100 mothers reported pain at some time. While it occurred primarily between the 3rd and 7th days, in some women it lasted for 6 weeks (Ziemer et al, 1990). Improper positioning of the infant and thrush are important causes of nipple pain. Treatment initiated by mothers often includes various creams, such as liquid Tylenol, baby oil, Oil of Olay, and Eucerin (Ziemer et al, 1990). These are not recommended forms of treatment. Be sure to ask nursing mothers who complain of nipple pain about measures they may have tried on their own to relieve the discomfort.

▼ Postpartum Depression

Symptoms of postpartum depression, a serious problem for many women, may appear at any time during the first year after the baby's birth. Not only is this depression a source of great distress for a new mother and her partner, but the irritability, fatigue, anger, worry, sadness, and anxiety that are present can also interfere with the mother's ability to respond and relate to her baby and other children. Thoughts of suicide and harming the baby may occur.

Postpartum depression should be distinguished from postpartum blues, a short-lived period of emotional lability that usually occurs toward the end of the first postpartum week and lasts only a day or two; and from postpartum psychosis, a condition involving unipolar depression, bipolar depression, or schizophrenia. Symptoms of postpartum psychosis include severe insomnia, hallucinations, agitation, and bizarre feelings or behavior. This condition requires immediate medical attention. Prompt identification and treatment of postpartum depression should be a high priority in any practice.

Questions about depression are not always part of the postpartum visit. For this reason and because postpartum depression may occur after the traditional 6-week postpartum visit, its occurrence is underestimated. Clinicians must be able to recognize the symptoms, respond to a woman's potential for harming herself or her baby, and make appropriate referrals to mental health professionals, support groups, and new mother groups. If the client seems unable to follow through with a referral, it is appropriate for the clinician to make an initial contact. Clinicians can also help a new mother mobilize sources of support and should call at intervals to see how she is doing. Since postpartum depression is likely to continue over a period of months, ongoing contact is beneficial.

Psychotropic medication is often indicated and may, at least initially, be preferable to psychotherapy because of the time it can take for psychotherapy to become effective.

About 10% of the time, postpartum depression is caused by postpartum thyroiditis, a transient condition that usually resolves spontaneously after 1 to 4 months. However, 1 in 4 women eventually develop a chronic hypothyroid condition. When postpartum depression occurs, thyroid testing should be requested to rule out a hyper- or hypothyroid state as the cause of symptoms. Medication to treat either the hyper- or hypothyroid state is often helpful while symptoms are present. Postpartum thyroiditis is likely to recur in subsequent pregnancies.

Appendix D lists helpful books for both clinicians and clients about postpartum depression.

▼ Incontinence

Newly delivered mothers may find they are incontinent of urine, flatus, or feces. Regrettably, few practitioners inquire about these problems. Many do not know that anal incontinence is a relatively common finding after delivery, particularly when forceps have been used to facilitate birth. It also occurs in noninstrumental deliveries. Since underreporting of incontinence is common, it is not surprising that few clinicians are aware that 1 out of 10 primiparas and 1 out of 5 multiparas who deliver vaginally may experience fecal urgency or the involuntary loss of flatus or feces. These symptoms even appear in women without obvious disruption of the rectal sphincter. Symptoms often disappear over time (Toglia & DeLancey, 1994).

All women should be asked about problems with incontinence, to avoid needless embarrassment and suffering. Reassure them that the symptoms usually disappear after 6 months. Encourage them to do Kegel exercises. If symptoms persist, a referral to a specialist is appropriate.

▼ Separated Symphysis

Peripartum separation of the pubic symphysis, although relatively rare, is a cause of significant maternal morbidity and, occasionally, long-term disability. It usually presents as significant pubic tenderness, with increased pain on turning in bed or ambulating. Pubic separation may be palpable. Often the client is not able to walk without assistance.

While a diagnosis can usually be made on the basis of symptoms, an x ray or ultrasound examination is often requested for confirmation. The size of the interpubic gap necessary for a diagnosis has not been determined. Suggestions of more than 8 mm and more than 10 mm have been made (Cibils, 1971; Hagen, 1974). The size of the gap has not been found to predict sequelae (Scriven, 1995).

Treatment of postpartum pubic separation involves a pelvic binder, analgesics, and ambulation using a walker. While most women have diminishing symptomatology over a period of weeks or months, symptoms may persist, necessitating use of a wheelchair. Surgery may be required.

▼ The Postpartum Visits

The 1- to 2-Week Postpartum Visit

The hallmark of ideal postpartum care is a series of home visits to check on the well-being of the newly delivered mother and her family. This approach is rarely available in the United States. In lieu of this ideal, telephone calls during the first week, followed by a visit to the clinician 1 or 2 weeks after the birth, are indicated. Unless problems exist, this visit can be primarily to evaluate the client's mental health; provide information and support; and ascertain the mother's feelings about the birth, her baby, the support available to her, and adjustments that have occurred within the family.

The 6-Week Checkup

Traditionally, the postpartum examination is scheduled approximately 6 weeks after delivery, but it may be performed any time between 4 and 8 weeks.

Perhaps the most important thing to remember about the 6-week visit is that it needs time if it is to be done well. Too often, only a breast and pelvic examination, and prescription of a method of birth control, are done. The 6-week visit should also be a time to review the pregnancy and birth experience, discuss problems, assess for depression, provide emotional support, answer questions, examine health risks, and consider whether or not a referral is indicated. The stance should be one of listening rather than giving advice.

Because of the time it takes to identify the issues that might be important to discuss, the client can fill out a postpartum history form before she is seen by the provider. (See Appendix X for sample questions.)

The Physical Examination

Examination of the Breasts

In addition to examining the breasts for masses, look for signs of nipple trauma if the client is breastfeeding. A good breast examination may be difficult if the breasts are full of milk. If the breast examination is inadequate, consider scheduling a return visit at a time when the breasts will be less full.

Be certain to discuss the importance of breast self-examination (BSE) at some time during the visit. New evidence indicating that breast tumors grow more rapidly in younger women (Kerlikowse, 1996) mandates that all women know the importance of this examination.

The Pelvic Examination

In addition to the regular components of a pelvic examination, the postpartum pelvic should include particular attention to the labia, the perineum, and the anus for signs of healing if lacerations occurred or an episiotomy was done. Pathology that may be noted includes a fistula and failure of a significant laceration to heal, resulting in disruption of the perineum. Referral to a gynecologist for evaluation may be indicated.

Occasionally, fusion of the upper portions of the labia will be noted. This can occur when bilateral, periurethral or labial lacerations have been minor and were left unrepaired. Usually this fusion causes no problem and should merely be noted.

A rectal examination, often "deferred" in childbearing women because of the discomfort and embarrassment associated with it, should always be performed at the postpartum examination to assess the integrity of the rectal sphincter. A rectal examination can also detect masses that are low in the pelvis and may have been missed on vaginal examination.

Laboratory Tests

Laboratory tests that may be appropriate at the postpartum examination include follow-up tests for conditions that were present during the pregnancy, and tests that are considered part of good care for women in general. Tests in the first category include a fasting blood sugar for women who were diagnosed with gestational diabetes to be certain that they are not true diabetics, and tests of thyroid function for women whose thyroid dosage changed as a result of the pregnancy. A fasting blood sugar of >140 mg/dL on two separate occasions confirms the diagnosis of non–insulin-dependent diabetes. Women with elevated fasting blood sugars should be referred to a physician.

Involvement of the Father or Partner

If a father or partner comes to the 6-week visit, try to arrange some time to determine his or her feelings and perceptions. If you did not have a chance prenatally to ask about the father or partner's childhood experiences, do it now. Be sure to ask if any parent or caretaker was an alcoholic or drug user. A referral to a parenting group, a support group, a mental health counselor, or sources of information may be in order for the father or partner.

Health Education

A variety of topics to improve health might be appropriate to discuss at the postpartum examination. One of the best guides to procedures and laboratory tests is *Clinician's Handbook of Preventive Services*, a 1994 publication of the U.S. Public Health Service. This book lists the recommendations of major authorities on 60 preventive care topics for children and adults. It can be ordered from the U.S. Government Printing Office, Box 371954, Pittsburgh, PA, 15250-7954, or from any of 24 U.S. Government Bookstores for $20 (GPO Stock #01700100496-1).

The book is part of an education kit that contains samples of three different preventive care flow sheets designed to serve as prompts for the health care provider; small, personal health care booklets for clients that summarize preventive health care practices and track care that has been received; samples of two types of reminder postcards; 16 kinds of self-sticking, colored "alert" notices to remind clinicians about certain aspects of a client's life (eg, smoking, alcohol use, high blood pressure, sun exposure, and elevated cholesterol); two preventive care timelines for display; and prevention prescriptions on which the clinician can write instructions for changes in behavior. This kit costs $57 (GPO Stock #01700100492-8).

Another helpful source of health education material is the Agency for Health Care Policy and Research (AHCPR), which publishes a set of documents on a variety of topics, including depression. The three documents available on each topic are *Clinical Practice Guidelines, A Quick Reference Guide for Clinicians* (a summary of the *Clinical Practice Guidelines)*, and a *Patient's Consumer Guide*. (The latter two documents are available free, as are some of the *Clinical Practice Guidelines.* To request a list of publications available, call AHCPR at 1-800-358-9295, or 410-381-3150 outside the United States.) Be sure to read the *Patient Consumer Guides* carefully for literacy level.

Breastfeeding

Women who are breastfeeding may appreciate information about leaking, breastfeeding while working, breastfeeding in public, support groups, and weaning. If a discussion about sexual activity and breastfeeding has not occurred, you might talk about the possibility of decreased lubrication, and also about the "let-down" reflex activated with orgasm. Breastfeeding mothers may wish to wear a bra or place a protective covering over the place of lovemaking. They may also wish to offer their partners a bit of breast milk, since many are curious about its taste.

Clinicians can help breastfeeding women who will be working outside the home anticipate a variety of reactions to the decision to work and breastfeed. Talk about possible responses should an unpleasant or inappropriate remark occur. See Box 4-3 for suggestions for women who anticipate joining or returning to the work force while breastfeeding.

Box 4-3. Suggestions for Breastfeeding Women Employed Outside the Home

1. Stay at home as long as possible.
2. Work part-time if possible.
3. Make some "practice runs"—a few hours away from the baby to anticipate problems.
4. Have an extra set of towels, an extra bra, and a change of clothes at the work site.
5. Take a quart of liquid to work and remember to drink it frequently.
6. Practice with a pump ahead of time so that you get used to it and the milk will let-down quickly.
7. If working full-time and manual expression or a manual pump is objectionable or does not work well, rent a dual hook-up electric pump to keep at work.
8. Find a place at work where you can feel comfortable and can have some privacy while you pump.
9. Have a backup place at work for pumping in case your first-choice place is not available.
10. If the baby will be in day care, be certain the day care provider is supportive of breastfeeding.
11. Arrive early at the day care provider's site so that you can nurse the baby right before going to work. This will help the baby settle down and allows time for talking with the daycare provider.

Clinicians also need to talk with women who have discontinued breastfeeding about their reasons for doing so as well as their feelings about stopping. While some will be relieved about changing to bottlefeeding, other women will be distressed, sad, and feel inadequate.

Birth Control

All women should be offered a method of birth control at the postpartum visit. Two particularly good books for clinicians are:

Hatcher, R.A., Trussell, J., Stewart, F., Stewart, G.K., Guest, F., Cates. W., Jr., & Policar, M.S. (1994). *Contraceptive Technology* (Rev. ed.). New York: Irvington.
Speroff, L., & Darney, P.D. (1996). *A Clinical Guide for Contraception* (2nd ed.). Baltimore: Williams and Wilkins.

Young adolescents are a particularly vulnerable group for repeat pregnancy. Despite thousands of programs in this country to prevent teenage pregnancy, the incidence of births to teenage girls in recent decades has not changed. Many intelligent and well-meaning adults have tried and failed to help young girls abstain from early intercourse or to use contraception effectively.

Most teenage girls *know* about contraception and how pregnancy occurs. But knowledge and behavior are only sometimes related. Most teenage pregnancy prevention programs fail to realize that teenage girls who are sexually active frequently lack the cognitive, interpersonal, and emotional skills to be successful contraceptors. A history of abuse, particularly sexual abuse, may be especially likely to influence a girl's ability to say "No" to sex or to use contraception effectively.

> *The onus of preventing a substantial portion of adolescent pregnancy must be located within the treatment field of child abuse and maltreatment. Attention must be paid to the long-term effects of abuse on development, self-esteem, and self-efficacy, including how the meaning of victimization will change and re-emerge at different developmental stages within the lives of adolescent girls (Boyer et al, 1991).*

Girls (and others) who have been sexually abused are often skilled at disassociation, able to "check out" of their bodies to avoid physical and psychic pain. Disassociation may become their way of moving through the world, of numbing themselves to feeling. If this happens, they may experience cognitive and motor dysfunction manifested in poor language skills and inability to follow directions or perform certain tasks—putting on a condom, for example. To a young girl who has experienced physical, sexual, or emotional abuse, either as an observer or as a victim, and who has been raised in poverty, lives without hope of bettering her life, and lacks self-confidence and self-esteem, it seems reasonable and logical to look for someone to love her. Why not a baby?

While multidisciplinary teams often work together to provide comprehensive care in a loving and sensitive manner, unfortunately this approach frequently doesn't help. No matter how caring the environment at a clinic or office, young adolescents frequently return home to an abusive environment. The focus of most teen pregnancy programs is young women, thus excluding a significant number of those contributing to the problem—adult men.

Successful family planning for young teenagers starts by recognizing that contraceptive decisions for young girls are complex. Clinicians must recognize the high incidence of physical, emotional, and sexual abuse in this society, and the likelihood that sexual abuse has occurred to any girl whose first sexual experience occurred before the age of 15 (Boyer & Fine, 1992). Clinicians should know that, in 70% of the births that occur to girls through age 18 in this country, adult men are the fathers. "How can young girls enforce abstinence or contraception upon adult men several years their senior . . . ?" (Oregon Pregnancy Prevention Taskforce, 1966) They must attend to the developmental tasks of adolescence and the worries and fears adolescent girls have about relationships, as well as the side effects of methods of birth control.

Access to social support programs that include job training and budgeting, an aggressive follow-up program, more frequent provider visits, and longer visits should be available. Clinicians may find it helpful to begin postpartum counseling by asking "What are some of the things you like to do? What do you want for yourself now and in the future? How does sex fit in? How does another baby fit in?"

Smoking

Many women who stop smoking while they are pregnant resume smoking in the months following delivery. Use the postpartum visit to reinforce the importance of a smoke-free environment for the client and for her children. Remind her of the link between parental smoking and lower respiratory illnesses (bronchitis, bronchiolitis, pneumonia); asthma; ENT problems; sudden infant death syndrome (SIDS); and meningococcal disease. Try the "30-second stop-smoking prompt": ". . . Don't smoke while holding your baby or while children are near. Keep your home and auto smoke free. Don't let others smoke around your children" (Oregon Health Division, 1996).

Be sure to screen for smoking at every visit. Realize that smoking cessation is a process accomplished over time and not likely to occur the first time that a clinician recommends quitting. Mark charts with a plainly visible sticker that identifies smoking clients. Ask the client if she would like to quit. If she responds affirmatively, ask "Why?" Knowing the reason the client wants to quit gives the clinician a chance to link symptoms or illnesses to smoking. Many clients benefit from a "quit date," a date set by the client for quitting and written by the clinician on a prescription pad. Refer to a local smoking cessation program when appropriate.

Discuss obstacles to quitting—previous failures, fear of weight gain, smoking by other family members, and unpleasant withdrawal symptoms. These may be minimized by reminding clients that most smokers need several tries before they succeed, that the average weight gain is 5 to 10 lb, that "No Smoking Zones" can be established, and that withdrawal symptoms are transient. Finally, have a system of follow-up for your clients who are willing to set quit dates (Cummings, 1995).

On the other hand, remember that it is not possible for every woman to stop smoking, even when she intellectually realizes that a child's health is at stake. The lives of many women have been and are filled with pain. They always deserve our gentleness and kindness.

Risks for the HIV Virus

The postpartum visit is an appropriate time to discuss the risks associated with sexual activity with multiple partners. Globally, more than one third of those infected with the human immunodeficiency virus (HIV) are women. The impact is greatest among women in central Africa, South America, Thailand, and southern India. In the United States, where the proportion of AIDS cases among females is 18% (CDC, 1995a), HIV rates are highest in California, Connecticut, Delaware, Florida, Georgia, Maryland, New Jersey, New York, Texas, Washington, D.C., Puerto Rico, and the Virgin Islands (CDC, 1995h). While HIV infection rates remain highest in the Northeastern United States, the greatest proportionate increases have occurred in the South and Midwest (CDC, 1995a).

The risk of infection from sexual intercourse can be decreased by practicing "safer sex." This means avoiding sex with high-risk partners; avoiding anal intercourse; using latex condoms when having sex with anyone other than a single, mutually-monogamous partner known to be HIV-negative; and limiting sexual relationships to those with a mutually-monogamous partner known to be HIV-negative.

Condom Use

Negotiating safer sex is a complex process. It involves recognizing that males usually dominate heterosexual relationships, and that a change in behavior from not using to using condoms will be difficult. For some women, the cost incurred by asking a partner to use a condom is too high. Loss of the relationship as well as loss of food, shelter, and even one's children or one's life, can be at stake.

If the client is known to you, you might begin a discussion of safer sex by returning to information about sexual practices obtained at the first prenatal visit. "I remember that you told me . . ." can be an opener. If the client is in a high-risk group for HIV and other sexually transmitted diseases, express your concern, then ask "What do you think about using condoms when you have sex?" You might continue with "Have you ever used one before?" "How did it go?" "Have you ever had a bad experience with a condom? Maybe it broke (or it interrupted lovemaking, or wouldn't stay on, or didn't taste good, or your partner said it was too tight, or he couldn't feel as well, or he didn't like having to pull out . . . ?)"

You might also begin a discussion of safer sex by asking "Have you talked with your partner about sexually transmitted diseases?" If not, you can ask "Would you see any problems with doing that?" or What do you think would happen if you started talking about them?" It might also be helpful to ask "What do you think other people should do in this situation?"

If the client does not have a current sexual partner, ask "What do you think might happen if you ask a new sexual partner to use a condom?"

Helpful facts about condoms include the kinds; brand names; what to look for on the label; how condoms vary in size, color, texture, taste, smell, thickness, and price; and where they are likely to be located in a store. This information can be obtained by purchasing a representative sample of condoms in the pharmacy section of a well-known grocery store. Examine the condoms with your client.

Counseling should include teaching how to put the condom on. A good way to teach a client the correct technique is to use a penis model. These can be obtained from a variety of catalog sources, but any penis-shaped object such as a cucumber, banana, or zucchini squash will do. After demonstrating the technique to the client, ask her to put the condom on the model herself. This will give her an opportunity to feel and smell the condom as well as to practice an effective technique that she can use herself or teach to her partner. Interjecting humor by blowing a condom up like a balloon and filling it with water may make it easier for the client to talk about it.

You might ask the client if she would like some help thinking of answers to common remarks partners have been known to make when the subject of condoms is initiated. Acknowledge that the first discussion about condom use is likely to be awkward and embarrassing. Condom use during sex with either a casual or a regular sexual partner is not a common practice in the United States. Ask the client what it might be like for her to bring up the subject. If she thinks she might have difficulty getting started, you might suggest she begin by talking about a television show she has seen in which one of the characters talked about using a condom. She might also talk about a newspaper article, a movie, a comment on a radio show, a billboard, a remark by a friend, or a pamphlet she brought from a clinic.

Common partner responses to suggestions about using condoms include: "They're not romantic."; "They decrease the feeling."; "They might break."; and "Don't you trust me?" If the client is unable to think of a reply, you might suggest the following responses:

"Let me show you how romantic they can be."
"AIDS isn't romantic either."
"Yes, condoms do break, but it's less than 1 time out of 100."
"It's not a matter of trust, it's a matter of health."
"You're not my first partner, and I want to be sure you are protected; I'm
    probably not your first partner, and I know you want to see me protected
    as well."

(See Appendix Y for additional suggestions.)

Prevention messages about sexually transmitted diseases need to be ongoing, as clients are not likely to stop engaging in risky practices immediately. Be direct with the information you want to convey. For example, when talking about condoms, you might say "You need to know three things about condoms:

they should be made of latex, they should be lubricated, and you must be certain of the expiration date." These messages must also be sensitive to the client's cultural or ethnic background, educational level, sexual identity, style of communication, and social skills.

All clinical encounters can be viewed as an opportunity to support behavioral change. These encounters must always consider the importance of men's power in sexual relationships, the tradition of female passivity in sexual matters, the custom of ignoring the needs and desires of women, and our legacy of thinking of sex as men do (ie, foreplay as a prelude to penis-in-vagina sex rather than as an alternative) (Taylor, 1995).

Weight Reduction

Most postpartum women have considerable weight to lose after having a baby. Unfortunately, most people find that losing weight is a difficult task. Maintaining the weight loss is even more difficult. The most useful approach to weight loss in clinical practice may be to identify obese clients most likely to medically benefit from a weight loss program, and to advise other clients about wise food choices.

Obesity is arbitrarily defined as a weight that is 120% or greater of desirable weight when a person's actual weight is divided by the desirable weight (as determined by an acceptable weight table). Those most at risk for obesity-related adverse health outcomes are women with a waist (measured at the umbilicus) to hip (measured at the greater trochanters) ratio above 0.8. Ratios higher than 0.8 reflect abdominal and/or visceral obesity and are associated with increased morbidity and mortality.

For women who want to lose weight, clinicians can emphasize the importance of eating "reasonable" amounts of a variety of healthy foods each day; encourage a regular program of exercise; and discuss the value of reading food labels. New U.S. Department of Agriculture regulations require that nutrition information appear on the labels of almost all foods. The labeling is useful; serving size is defined and, in many cases, is more reflective of the amount of food a person is likely to consume than in previous labeling. Information about nutrients that people are concerned about today (eg, saturated fat, cholesterol, and fiber) is included.

Recent nutrition education programs tend to focus on decreasing the amount of fat and saturated fat in the American diet. But emphasizing fat alone fails to tell the whole story. Many Americans feel that decreasing fat in their diet gives them license to eat as much as they want of other foods, which can lead to a high-calorie diet. Starchy foods are fattening.

Unfortunately, despite recent research suggesting that the obese woman is not always responsible for her obese state, many practitioners continue to believe that losing weight is merely a matter of willpower. Practitioners would do well to recognize that the cause of obesity is multifactorial. Not only behavioral factors (physical activity and food choices), but strong genetic influences, medical illness, and medications contribute to the problem of overweight. Clinicians might think about the words of a woman who, by height and weight, is categorized as "morbidly obese."

> *I do eat. I also work, sing, paint, write, volunteer in the community, help my neighbors, garden, walk the dog, love my husband, take care of and love my kids, spend money, call my mother, kiss my granddaughter and have parties once in a while. . . . So why does society want to change a cow into a deer? Why did I try the same things for 35 years myself? I guess I forgot about the important things*

in life and about people like my Uncle Gene. With the kindest heart in the world, he was adored and admired by everyone who knew him until the day he died. I've never met anyone fatter. . . . We are who we are. I happen to be more than some would want me to be, but that does not make me less (Madrigal, 1995).

A new dietary reference term on food labels is the Daily Value (DV). It is made up of two different sets of references, the Daily Reference Value (DRV), and the Reference Daily Intake (RDI). A reference point rather than a recommended amount, DRV identifies the percent of the daily value that one serving of the food provides. Table 4-1 contains the DRVs for energy-producing nutrients, based on 2000 calories per day.

The term "RDI" is being used to replace the term "U.S. RDA" in hopes of avoiding the confusion that has occurred between "RDAs" (Recommended *Dietary* Allowances, set by the National Academy of Sciences, and updated as new knowledge warrants) and "U.S. RDAs" (Recommended *Daily* Allowances). Reference Daily Intakes (RDIs) still serve as a reference value for essential vitamins, minerals, and protein (Food and Drug Administration, 1993).

Clients not accustomed to reading labels often appreciate help in this area. Try removing labels from cans and packages. Place them in plastic casings in a 3-ring binder to show to clients, selecting labels that illustrate the points you wish to make.

Calcium

Women of childbearing age should consume 1200 mg of calcium daily. While the body absorbs calcium equally well from calcium carbonate, calcium lactate, and calcium gluconate, the least expensive supplementary source of calcium is TUMS, which contains 200 mg of calcium carbonate per tablet.

High doses of calcium carbonate can cause constipation and flatulence. While calcium gluconate is less constipating, it is considerably more expensive. A chelated calcium product is also more expensive and has no advantage over a nonchelated product. Bone meal and dolomite as calcium sources should be

TABLE 4-1. DRVs for the Energy-Producing Nutrients (fat, carbohydrate, protein, and fiber) Based on 2000 Calories a Day for Adults

Food Component	DRV
Fat	65 g
Saturated fatty acids	20 g
Cholesterol	300 mg
Total carbohydrate	300 g
Fiber	25 g
Sodium	2400 mg
Potassium	3500 mg
Protein (nonpregnant adults)	50 g
Protein (nursing mothers)	65 g

(From Food and Drug Administration. (1993). Focus on food labeling (Special Report). *FDA Consumer.* Washington, D.C.: Department of Health and Human Services.)

avoided as they may be contaminated with lead. Note that 1 cup of plain yogurt contains twice as much calcium (415 mg) as 1 tablet of Tums; 1 cup of milk contains 1½ times as much (300 mg).

Depression

Depression (separate from postpartum depression) may be a recurrent theme in the lives of women. It is important to identify depression because a depressed woman may be unable to respond to her baby's or children's cues, neglect her children, be unable to relate to a partner, or commit suicide. It is also important to talk with women about depression because many women do not know they are depressed and can benefit from psychotherapy, behavioral therapy, or newer psychotropic drugs.

Clinicians should remember that not only is depression recurrent, it is associated with significant morbidity and even mortality. Since approximately 15% of people who are depressed commit suicide, depression should be viewed as a potentially fatal illness. Depressed women deserve to be identified and offered appropriate therapy.

In the past, nursing has focused almost exclusively on psychodynamic and behavioral theories of mental illness. However, recent research has demonstrated that many cases of depression have a biologic basis, a deficiency in amine neurotransmitters which, among other things, lowers the level of serotonin, a mood regulator, in the brain. A relatively new category of drugs, the selective serotonin reuptake inhibitors (SSRIs), increase serotonin. Fluoxetine (Prozac), paroxidine (Paxil), and sertraline (Zoloft) are commonly used SSRIs. While many clinicians are not prepared to prescribe these drugs themselves, referral to someone who can evaluate the client to determine if their use is appropriate is often indicated.

Clinicians need to be knowledgeable about these drugs so that the women who take them can receive appropriate support should they have questions or concerns. For example, women taking one of these drugs may ask how long it takes for a response to occur; when is it appropriate to consider changing drugs; and how long therapy should be continued once depressive symptoms are relieved. Knowing that it takes 6 weeks or longer to know who will respond; that in some ways the SSRIs are like NSAIDs and a person may respond well to one drug and not to another; and that drug therapy should probably be continued for 9 to 12 months, is helpful.

Use of medication to treat depression is objectionable to some clinicians because of personal biases that blame a woman for not being able to "pull herself out of it," and the implication that a woman who depends on a drug for her mental well-being is weak. These beliefs are not only wrong, they are destructive. Some health care providers may have been trained to view psychological problems exclusively from a psychosocial perspective; may be unfamiliar with psychotropic drugs; or may prefer not to use medication because, until recently, the only drugs available were the tricyclic antidepressants and monoamine oxidase inhibitors. These drugs have many side effects, and clients often discontinue using them.

Short-term therapy with psychotropic drugs is likely to be helpful in 65% to 80% of people who take the medication. The risks of these drugs to the baby when mothers are breastfeeding have not been studied, so their use must be weighed against the benefits. Clearly, however, there are times when their use should take precedence over breastfeeding. Psychotropic drugs can also benefit women with dysthymia (the chronically unhappy), bulimia, and premenstrual dysphoria disorder.

Because depression is not always biologic, psychotherapy alone or in combination with an appropriate drug may be in order. Unfortunately, psychotherapy may be more expensive than pharmacotherapy and may not be available to women, even with health insurance.

Bipolar Disorder

Lithium prophylaxis for postpartum women with a history of bipolar disorder has been recommended to prevent relapse, estimated to occur in 20% to 50% of these women (Cohen et al, 1995). Concern, of course, is for the significant amount of the drug secreted into breast milk. Its effect on nursing babies is not known. The benefits of lithium may be acceptable despite the risk. Certainly, some women will choose to give their babies formula so that they do not have to worry about lithium in their breast milk.

The decision to give up breastfeeding in favor of psychoactive drugs can be difficult for some health care providers to support. Yet women have a right to be free of the pain and suffering that a mental disease imposes. Health care providers must act in a responsible and professional manner in letting women know their options.

Immunizations

The postpartum period is an opportune time to immunize against rubella and varicella because most women wish to refrain from a subsequent pregnancy for at least 3 months, the period of time to avoid pregnancy when a live-virus vaccine is administered. Side effects of rubella vaccine include a slight fever, rash, enlarged lymph nodes, and arthralgias 3 to 25 days after receiving the vaccine. Those with a history of an anaphylactic reaction to neomycin should not be immunized against rubella, as neomycin is found in this vaccine.

Two subcutaneous doses of varicella vaccine given 4 to 8 weeks apart confer immunity to 94% of those receiving the vaccine. Seroconversion lasts 7 to 13 years in 80% of cases. Side effects include tenderness and erythema at the injection site (25%), and a generalized maculopapular rash within 1 month of the injection (5%) (Medical Letter, 1995).

The postpartum period is also an excellent time to catch up on other immunizations. Vaccines that should be offered include tetanus-diphtheria (Td); polio, if the series was incomplete during childhood; hepatitis B (now recommended for everyone); and mumps, if women have not had the disease or been vaccinated. Every adult needs tetanus vaccine because any wound can become contaminated with tetanus. Tetanus vaccine is given in combination with diphtheria, a disease not well-known in developed countries. However, diphtheria struck 80,000 people in Russia, and protection is prudent. Adults should be immunized against tetanus every ten years. Find a way to help clients remember their 10-year anniversary, perhaps by using the ages 25, 35, 45, and so on as a reminder.

Hepatitis B vaccine should be given in the deltoid muscle rather than in the buttocks because of increased immunogenicity when administered in the arm. Two intramuscular doses are given 4 weeks apart, and the third dose is given 5 months after the second (American College of Physicians, 1993). When a subsequent antibody titre is positive, protection is thought to last 7 to 10 years. Screening with the hepatitis B surface antibody test should be done before a booster is given.

Since 1989, a second dose of the measles–mumps–rubella vaccine has been recommended for adults who were vaccinated against measles before 1979 because people vaccinated before 1979, when a new "stabilizer" was added, have a higher risk of getting measles. People born before 1956 are considered immune to measles because of the very high likelihood that they have had the disease.

Hepatitis A vaccine is now available and should be offered to anyone who wants this immunity, particularly travelers.

Cancer

Counseling about risk for cancer is often appropriate at the postpartum checkup. Inherited forms of cancer (10%–15% of cancer cases) are classified as hereditary cancer syndromes, in which the risk for developing a specific form of cancer may be almost 90%; hereditary preneoplastic syndromes, in which cancer occurs as a secondary effect of the disorder; and familial cancers, in which cancer occurs in families at higher than expected rates.

"Although any form of cancer has the potential of being familial, the most common familial cancers are those of the breast, ovary, colon, endometrium, lymphoid and hemopoetic tissue, and brain" (Schneider, 1994). A significant family history of cancer includes two or more relatives with the same or related cancers; earlier onset than is typical for that cancer; rare cancers; bilateral disease in paired organs (eg, tumors in both breasts, eyes, kidneys, or ovaries); and multiple, primary cancers (two or more different cancers in one person).

All women should be taught and encouraged to perform SBE. Recent evidence showing that breast tumors in younger women can grow rapidly in less than a year reinforces the need to encourage all women to perform this monthly examination (Kerliwoske, 1996). Women also should know the recommended ages for initial and follow-up mammograms, and they should be encouraged to share this information with female friends and family members.

Guidelines issued in 1989 by the National Cancer Institute and other medical organizations recommended a baseline mammogram between the ages of 35 and 40 and mammography plus a breast examination by a clinician every 1 to 2 years between the ages of 40 and 49. However, in 1993 the National Cancer Institute withdrew its support for screening women aged 40 to 49 because the supposedly dense breast tissue in women of this age group makes radiographic interpretation difficult; in addition, no benefit was discernable.

A recent analysis of the statistics used in the 1989 report concluded:

> The data strongly suggest that women aged 40 to 49 should be advised to be screened every year rather than every two years. Screening by mammography and clinical breast examination, if performed properly, can be expected to reduce the death rate from breast cancer for women in this decade by at least 25% to 30% (Kopans, 1996, p. 1289).

Another article of support appeared in 1995:

> We support the routine use of mammographic screening for all women aged 40 to 49 years because we interpret the evidence as indicating a high probability of benefit. Currently, more than 10,000 deaths occur per year in the United States among women who developed breast cancer between the ages of 40 and 49, and 30% of the years of life lost to breast cancer are among these women. Because the probable benefit of screening involves at least a 20% reduction in deaths from breast cancer, thousands of lives are probably lost each year because of indecision and inaction. It seems much more prudent to endorse screening now and risk the unlikely subsequent determination that the effort was ineffective, than to withhold screening until it is determined whether "proof" will be obtained and risk the loss of so many women in the prime of life (Sickles & Kopans, 1995).

Table 4-2 estimates breast cancer risk for women by age. Data were taken from the National Cancer Institute's Surveillance, Epidemiology, and End Results (SEER) Program, 1975–1988. Women with a first-degree family history of breast cancer before age 50 should have an annual mammogram after the age of 30 (Burke, 1993).

At the postpartum visit, clinicians should also counsel clients who have hereditary neoplastic syndromes or familial cancers about the need for follow-up by a specialist. If a woman has two first-degree relatives who have had ovarian cancer, the National Institutes of Health have recommended annual recto-vaginal-pelvic examination, CA-125 determinations, and transvaginal ultrasound until age 35 (earlier, if childbearing is completed) when a prophylactic, bilateral oophorectomy is recommended.

A family history of polyposis requires colonoscopy every 3 to 5 years after the age of 18. If two or more first-degree relatives have had ovarian cancer, the client is at very high risk for one of three autosomal dominant hereditary ovarian cancer syndromes. Women with a first-degree family history of colon cancer, especially if it has occurred in two or more relatives before the age of 40, should also have colonoscopy every 3 to 5 years after the age of 40, and need annual hemoccult tests in their 30s. Some clinicians recommend annual screening before the age of 40 (Burke, 1993). For a few families, predisposition testing can provide information about cancer susceptibility.

Clinicians should also discuss cancer prevention with their clients. Skin cancer is one of the hazards of exposure to sunlight. Those most at risk have a family history of skin cancer or have sensitive skin (ie, those who always burn on exposure to the sun or who tan never or only slightly). Regular use of a sunscreen with a sun protection factor of 15 for the first 18 years of life can significantly decrease a person's lifetime risk of developing nonmelanoma skin cancer. Instruct clients to reapply sunscreen after swimming or sweating. Indoor sunlamps, tanning parlors, and tanning pills should be discouraged. Unfortunately, few teenagers always use sunscreen, and an alarming number—33% in one study—never use it. This same study reported that 33% of girls under the age of 16, and 56% of the 18-year-old girls, had been to a tanning salon at least once (Banks et al, 1992).

Self-examination of the skin should occur monthly and can be conducted with the monthly SBE. The skin examination should include:

- Examining the front and back of the body in a mirror
- Raising the arms and examining each side
- Bending the elbows to look at forearms, upper arms, and palms of the hand
- Sitting to look at the backs of the legs and feet, the soles of the feet, and the spaces between the toes
- Using a hand mirror to examine the back of the neck and the scalp (American Cancer Society, 1993).

Heart Disease

Screening for heart disease has not been common in women, probably because of the prevailing notion that heart disease is mainly a problem for men. Yet heart disease is the number one killer of women. While 1 out of 8 women will die from breast cancer, 1 out of 2 women will die from heart disease.

The risk factors for cardiac disease in women are the same as in men:

Smoking
High blood pressure
Diabetes

TABLE 4-2. Percent Developing Invasive Breast Cancer Before a Specified Age (Z), Given Free of Invasive Cancer at Current Age (Y) in SEER Areas, Women, All Races, 1987–1988

Current age (Years)	Develop cancer by age (Z), %									
	10	20	30	40	50	60	70	80	90	Eventually
0	0.00	0.00	0.04	0.46	1.99	4.24	7.35	10.39	12.10	12.57
10		0.00	0.04	0.46	2.01	4.29	7.44	10.51	12.24	12.72
20			0.04	0.47	2.02	4.30	7.46	10.55	12.29	12.76
30				0.43	1.99	4.29	7.47	10.57	12.32	12.80
40					1.58	3.91	7.13	10.28	12.04	12.53
50						2.41	5.74	9.01	10.83	11.33
60							3.59	7.10	9.07	9.62
70								4.13	6.45	7.08

(From Feuer, E.J., Wun, L-M. Boring, C.C., Flanders, W.D., Timmel, M.J., & Tong, T. (1993). The lifetime risk of developing breast cancer. *Journal of the National Cancer Institute, 85*, 894.)

High levels of low-density lipoprotein (LDL), and low levels of HDL-cholesterol (<35 mg/dL)

A family history of premature coronary heart disease (CHD).

A family history of a heart attack in one first-degree relative, or two second-degree relatives, before the age of 55 in men and 65 in women, increases risk. (Disease in first-degree relatives is more significant than with other relatives.) If the client is young, her parents may not be old enough to have developed CHD. In this case, be certain to inquire about a history of CHD in grandparents.

Preventive care guidelines recently issued by the American College of Physicians state:

> *Screening for total cholesterol levels is not recommended for . . . women (younger than 45 years of age) unless the history or physical examination suggests a familial lipoprotein disorder or at least two other characteristics increase the risk for coronary heart disease (American College of Physicians, 1996, p. 516).*

Box 4-4 illustrates the normal cholesterol lipoprotein profile.

Referrals

The postpartum visit is an opportune time to suggest a referral for additional help with problem areas. Referrals that might be appropriate at the postpartum visit include:

- A stop-smoking program
- An anger-control program
- Parenting programs
- Support groups
- Counseling or therapy
- Medical evaluation and treatment
  - High blood pressure
  - Abnormal laboratory tests
  - Thyroid enlargement
  - Unresolved incontinence (after 6 months)

Sometimes it seems that the people most likely to refrain from attending parenting classes are those most likely to need assistance. It is hard to know a good way to tell a mother that you think her ability to parent is lacking. You might try talking about the stress that a new baby brings to a family and then discuss parenting programs in terms of their focus on helping new parents deal with stress. In lieu of a referral to a parenting group, give one or two pamphlets about parenting issues to clients when you say goodbye at the postpartum visit.

Box 4-4. The Normal Cholesterol/Lipoprotein Profile

Total cholesterol:	Less than 200 mg/dL
HDL-cholesterol:	Greater than 50 mg/dL
LDL-cholesterol:	Less than 130 mg/dL
Triglycerides:	Less than 250 mg/dL

The Learning Curve has three ¾ × 9-inch fliers that come shrink-wrapped in packs of 100. The two-sided fliers ("Ten things to do before yelling or hitting" and "Think before you spank") are $8 per pack. The single-sided fliers ("Toilet mastery," "Separation," and "Shopping with children") are $7.50 per pack. A pamphlet, "Help your baby grow and learn: Ten tips for new parents," is priced according to quantity purchased (15 to 24 each). All are written at an 8th-grade reading level and are available from Learning Curve, 4614 Prospect Avenue, #421, Cleveland, OH. 44103-4314, 1-800-795-9295; fax: 216-881-7177. (Shipping and handling are extra.)

Support groups provide valuable supportive emotional care for women in a variety of circumstances. Since the health care provider may have minimal time available to discuss emotional responses to a new baby, or medical problems with a psychological component, participation in a support group may help a new mother work through her feelings and problems. Increased knowledge about the problem, concern, or feeling may facilitate adaptation to the new situation.

Health care providers need to learn about community support groups. Clients appreciate information about a group's philosophy, meeting times, location, and cost. Be sure to ask clients to give you feedback about the quality of any support group they attend.

Support groups that might be appropriate for a new mother or for a woman with a variety of circumstances include:

New mothers
Breastfeeding
Sexual abuse
Domestic violence
Children of alcoholic parents
Alcoholics Anonymous or Al-Anon

▼ Conclusion

The postpartum visit, while often considered to be routine and boring, can help a new mother feel good about herself. Since few abnormalities are likely to be found on physical examination, much of the visit can be spent assessing emotional well-being and helping the client evaluate her support system and establish goals for the future. The postpartum visit, therefore, is important and worthwhile.

At times, you as the clinician may feel that working with the client has felt like a gift. At other times, helplessness, anger, and frustration will prevail. Still, if at all times you care for women and their families with patience, compassion, thoughtfulness, and hope, you will influence many lives for the better.

References

▼ References

Addiction Counseling Certification Board of Oregon. (1995, May). Methcathinone. *ACCBO News.*

Adler, A.I., & Olscamp, A. (1995). Toxic "sock" syndrome: Bezoar formation and pancreatitis associated with iron deficiency anemia. *Western Journal of Medicine, 163,* 480–482.

Agency for Toxic Substances and Disease Registry. (1992). *Case studies in environmental medicine: Taking an exposure history.* Atlanta: U.S. Department of Health & Human Services.

Agnoli, F. (1994). Group B streptococcus: Perinatal considerations, *Journal of Family Practice, 39,* 171–177.

Alpert, E.J. (1995). Violence in intimate relationships and the practicing internist: New "disease" or new agenda? *Annals of Internal Medicine, 123,* 774–781.

American College of Obstetricians and Gynecologists. (1996). Hypertension in pregnancy (ACOG Technical Bulletin No. 219). Washington, D.C.: American College of Obstetricians and Gynecologists.

American College of Obstetricians and Gynecologists. (1993). Hemoglobinopathies in pregnancy (ACOG Technical Bulletin No. 185). Washington, D.C.: American College of Obstetricians and Gynecologists.

American College of Obstetricians and Gynecologists. (1990). Management of isoimmunization in pregnancy. (ACOG Technical Bulletin No. 148). Washington, D.C.: American College of Obstetricians and Gynecologists.

American College of Obstetricians and Gynecologists. (1987). Antenatal diagnosis of genetic disorders (ACOG Technical Bulletin No. 108). Washington, D.C.: American College of Obstetricians and Gynecologists.

American College of Physicians. (1996). Guidelines for using serum cholesterol, high-density lipoprotein cholesterol, and triglyceride levels as screening tests for preventing coronary heart disease in adults. *Annals of Internal Medicine, 124,* 515–517.

American Medical Association. (1994). *Drug evaluations annual (1994).* Washington, D.C.: American Medical Association.

Bachman, J.W., Heise, R.H., Naessens, J.M., & Timmerman, M.G. (1993). A study of various tests to detect asymptomatic urinary tract infections in an obstetric population, *Journal of the American Medical Association, 270,* 1974.

Banks, B.A., Silverman, Schwartz, R.H., & Tunnessen, W.W. (1992). Attitudes of teenagers toward sun exposure. *Pediatrics, 89,* 40–42.

Bowen, L.A. (1994). Trauma and pregnancy, *Clinician Reviews, 4*(3), 49+.

Boyer, D., & Fine, D. (1992). Sexual abuse as a factor in adolescent pregnancy and child maltreatment. *Family Planning Perspectives, 24*(1), 4–11.

Boyer, D., Fine, D., & Killpack, S. (1991). What is teen pregnancy? *WACSAP Newsletter, 16*(1), 6.

Brace, R.A., & Wolff, R.J. (1989). Normal amniotic fluid volume changes throughout pregnancy. *American Journal of Obstetrics and Gynecology,161,* 382. Burke, W. (1993). The non-routine "routine" family history. *Genetics Northwest, 8*(4), 2–5.

Burlbaw, J. (1996). Intrauterine growth restriction. *OB-GYN Ultrasound Today, 2*(3), 25–36.

Burtin, P., Taddio, A., Ariburnu, O., Einarson, T.R., & Koren, G. (1995). Safety of metronidazole in pregnancy: A meta-analysis. *American Journal of Obstetrics and Gynecology, 172,* 525–529.

Busch, W., & Himes, P. (1995). Maternal serum screening for chromosome disorders and open neural tube defects. *Genetics Northwest, 10*(2 & 3), 4–6.

Centers for Disease Control and Prevention. (1991). Weapon-carrying among high school students: United States, 1990. *Morbidity and Mortality Weekly Report, 40,* 681–684.

Centers for Disease Control and Prevention. (1993a). Reported vaccine-preventable diseases: United States, 1993, and the childhood immunization initiative. *Morbidity and Mortality Weekly Report, 43,* 57–60.

174 ▼ References

Centers for Disease Control and Prevention. (1993b). Jin Bu Huan toxicity in children: Colorado. *Morbidity and Mortality Weekly Report, 42*, 633–635.

Centers for Disease Control and Prevention. (1993c). Lead poisoning associated with use of traditional ethnic remedies: California, 1991–1992. *Morbidity and Mortality Weekly Report, 42*, 521–524.

Centers for Disease Control and Prevention. (1995a). First 500,000 AIDS cases: United States, 1995. *Morbidity and Mortality Weekly Report, 44*, 849–853.

Centers for Disease Control and Prevention. (1995b). Increasing morbidity and mortality associated with abuse of methamphetamine: United States, 1991–1994. *Morbidity and Mortality Weekly Report, 44*, 882–886.

Centers for Disease Control and Prevention. (1995c). Poverty and infant mortality—United States, 1988. *Morbidity and Mortality Weekly Report, 44*, 922–927.

Centers for Disease Control and Prevention. (1995d). Prevention and control of influenza: Recommendations of the advisory committee on immunization practices (ACIP). *Morbidity and Mortality Report, 44*(RR-3), 5.

Centers for Disease Control and Prevention. (1995e). U.S. Public Health Service recommendations for human immunodeficiency virus counseling and voluntary testing for pregnant women. *Morbidity and Mortality Weekly Report, 44*(RR-7), 1–14.

Centers for Disease Control and Prevention. (1995f). Self-treatment with herbal and other plant-derived remedies: Rural Mississippi, 1993. *Morbidity and Mortality Weekily Report, 44*, 204–207.

Centers for Disease Control and Prevention. (1995g). Anticholinergic poisoning associated with herbal tea. *Morbidity and Mortality Weekly Report, 44*, 193–195.

Centers for Disease Control and Prevention. (1995h). AIDS map. *Morbidity and Mortality Weekly Report, 44*, 719.

Centers for Disease Control and Prevention. (1996a). Progress toward elimination of neonatal tetanus: Egypt, 1988–1994. *Morbidity and Mortality Weekly Report, 45*(4), 89–92.

Centers for Disease Control and Prevention. (1996b). Prevention of perinatal Group B streptococcal disease: A public health perspective. *Morbidity and Mortality Weekly Report, 45*(RR-7), 1–24.

Centers for Disease Control and Prevention. (1996). Outbreak of primary and secondary syphilis: Baltimore City, Maryland, 1995. Editorial Note. *Morbidity and Mortality Weekly Report, 45*(8), 166–169.

Chapman, L.L. (1992). Expectant fathers' roles during labor and birth. *JOGNN, 21*, 114–120.

Chasnoff, I.J., Landress, H.L., & Barrett, M.E. (1990). The prevalence of illicit-drug or alcohol use during pregnancy and discrepancies in mandatory reporting in Pinellas County, Florida. *The New England Journal of Medicine, 322*, 1202–1206.

Cibils, L.A. (1971). Rupture of the symphysis pubis. *Obstetrics and Gynecology, 38*, 407.

Cohen, L.S., Sichel, D.A., Robertson, L.M., Heckscher, E., & Rosenbaum, J.F. (1995). Postpartum prophylaxis for women with bipolar disorder. *American Journal of Psychiatry, 152*, 1641–1645.

Collaborative Group on Preterm Birth. (1993). Multicenter randomized, controlled trial of a preterm birth prevention program. *American Journal of Obstetrics and Gynecology, 169u*, 352–366.

Committee on Infectious Diseases and Committee on Fetus and Newborn. (1992). Guidelines for prevention of early onset group B streptococcal sepsis, *Pediatrics, 90*, 775–780.

Connor, E.M., Sperling, R.S., Gelber, R., Kiselev, P., Scott, G., O'Sullivan, M.J., VanDyke, R., Bey, M., Shearer, W., Jacobson, R.L., Jimenez, E., O'Neill, E., Bazin, B., Delfraissy, J-F., Culnane, M., Coombs, R., Elkins, M., Moye, J., Stratton, P., & Balsley, J. (1994). Reduction of maternal-infant transmission of human immunodeficiency virus type 1 with zidovudine treatment. *New England Journal of Medicine, 331*:1173–80.

Cooksey, N.R. (1995). Pica and olfactory craving of pregnancy: How deep are the secrets? *Birth, 22*, 129–137.

Cummings, S.R. (1995, August 24). Helping Smokers Quit. Talk given at *Essentials of Primary Care: A Core Curriculum for Practice in the Managed Care Era*, Squaw Creek, North Lake Tahoe, CA. Presented by Division of Internal Medicine, University of California at San Francisco School of Medicine.

Cunningham, F.G., Leveno, K.J. (1995). Childbearing among older women: The message is cautiously optimistic. *New England Journal of Medicine, 333*, 1002–1004.

Cunningham, F.G., MacDonald, P.C., Gant, N.F., Leveno, K.J., & Gilstrap, L.C., III. (1993). *Williams Obstetrics* (19th ed.). Norwalk, CT: Appleton & Lange.

Cutforth, R., & MacDonald, C.B. (1966). Heart sounds and murmurs in pregnancy. *American Heart Journal, 71*, 741–747.

Dacus, J.V., Meyer, N.L., & Sibai, B.M. (1995). How preconception counseling improves pregnancy outcome. *Contemporary OB/GYN, 40*(6), 111+.

Doak, C.C., Doak, L.G., & Root, J.H. (1996). *Teaching patients with low literacy skills* (2nd ed.). Philadelphia: J.B. Lippincott.

Dumars, K.W., Boehm, C., Eckman, J.R., Giardina, P. J., Lane, P.A., & Shafer, F.E. for the Council of Regional Networks for Genetic Services (CORN). (1996). Practical guide to the diagnosis of thalassemia. *American Journal of Medical Genetics, 62*, 29–37.

Eisenberg, D.M., Kessler, R.C., Foster, C., Norlock, F.E., Calkins, D.R., & Delblanco, T.L. (1993). Unconventional medicine in the United States. *New England Journal of Medicine, 328*, 246–252.

Ende, J., Rockwell, S., & Glasgow, M. (1984). The sexual history in general medicine practice. *Archives of Internal Medicine, 144*, 558–561.

Enkin, M., Keirse, M.J.N.C., Renfrew, M., & Neilson, J. (1995). *A guide to effective care in pregnancy and childbirth.* New York: Oxford University Press.

Etherington, I.J., & James, D.K. (1993). Reagent strip testing of antenatal urine specimens for infection. *British Journal of Obstetrics and Gynecology, 100*, 806–808.

Fairley, C.K., Smoleniec, J.S., Caul, O.E., & Miller, E. (1995). Observational study of effect of intrauterine transfusions on outcome of fetal hydrops after parovirus B19 infection. *Lancet, 346*, 1335–1337.

Farkas, C. S., Glenday, P.G., O'Connor, P.J., & Schmeltzer, J. (1987). Evaluation of the readability of prenatal health education materials. *Canadian Journal of Public Health, 78*, 374–378.

Ferenczy, A. (1995). Epidemiology and clinical pathophysiology of condylomata acuminata. *American Journal of Obstetrics and Gynecology, 172*, 1331–1339.

Feuer, E.J., Wun, L-M, Boring, C.C., Flanders, W.D., Timmel, M.J., & Tong, T. (1993). The lifetime risk of developing breast cancer. *Journal of the National Cancer Institute, 85*, 892–897.

Fish, C. (1988). Woman abuse: The role of the health care provider. *American Journal of Gynecologic Health, 3*, (3), 48–57.

Foster, J.C., & Smith, H.L. (1996). Use of the Cytobrush for Papanicolau smear screens in pregnant women. *Journal of Nurse-Midwifery, 41*, 211–217.

Fullerton, J.T., Wallace, H.M., Concha-Garcia, S. (1993). Development and translation of an English-Spanish dual-language instrument addressing access to prenatal care for the border-dwelling Hispanic women of San Diego County. *Journal of Nurse-Midwifery, 38*, 45–50.

Gall, S.A. (1995). Immunizations for patients and personnel. *Contemporary OB/GYN, 40*, 29+.

Gazmararanian, J.A., Lazorick, J., Spitz, A.M., Ballard, T.J., Saltzman, L.E., & Marks, J.S. (1996). Prevalence of violence against pregnant women. *Journal of the American Medical Association, 275*, 1915–1920.

Ghidini, A. (1996). Idiopathic fetal growth restriction: A pathophysiologic approach. *Obstetrical and Gynecological Survey, 51*, 376–382.

Gibbs, R.S., & Sweet, R.L. (1994). Maternal and fetal infections. In R.K. Creasy & R. Resnik (Eds.), *Maternal-fetal medicine: Principles and practice.* Philadelphia: W.B. Saunders.

Graham, H. (1988). Health education. In A. McPherson (Ed.), *Women's problems in general practice.* New York: Oxford University Press.

Greenland, V.C., Delke, I., & Minkoff, H.L. (1989). Vaginally administered cocaine overdose in a pregnant woman. *American Journal of Obstetrics and Gynecology, 74*, 476–477.

Gribble, R.K., Meier, Paul, R., & Berg, R.L. (1995). The value of urine screening for glucose at each prenatal visit, *Obstetrics and Gynecology, 86*, 405–410.

Hanford Health Information Network. (1994). Genetic effects and birth defects from radiation exposure. (A collaboration of 3 states and 9 Indian nations. HHIN Resource Center: 1-800-959-7660).

Harlap, S., & Shiono, P.H. (1980). Alcohol, smoking, and incidence of spontaneous abortions in the first and second trimester. *Lancet, 2,* 173–176.

Helton, A.S., McFarlane, J., & Anderson, E.T. (1987). Battered and pregnant: A prevalence study. *American Journal of Public Health, 77,* 1337–1339.

Henriksen, T.B., Hedegaard, M., Secher, N.J., & Wilcox, A.J. (1995). Standing at work and preterm delivery, *British Journal of Obstetrics and Gynecology, 102,* 198–206.

Johnson, M.J., Petri, M., Witter, F.R., & Repke, J.T. (1995). Evaluation of preterm delivery in a systemic lupus erythematosus pregnancy clinic, *Obstetrics and Gynecology, 86,* 396–399.

Katz, V.L., Kuller, J.A., McMahon, M.J., Warren, M.A., & Wells, S.R. (1995). Varicella during pregnancy: Maternal and fetal effects. *Western Journal of Medicine, 163,* 446–450.

Kerlikowske, L. (1996) *Journal of the American Medical Association, 275,*

Kirsch, I.S., Jungeblut, A., Jenkins, L., & Kolstad, A. (1993). *Adult literacy in America: A first look at the results of the National Adult Literacy Survey.* Washington, D.C.: U.S. Government Printing Office.

Kopans, D.B. (1995). Mammography screening and the controversy concerning women aged 40 to 49. *Radiologic Clinics of North America, 33,* 1273–1290.

Laros, R. K., Jr. (1994). Maternal hematologic disorders. In R. Creasy and R.K. Resnik (Eds.), *Maternal-Fetal Medicine: Principles and Practice.* Philadelphia: W.B. Saunders.

Leiner, S., & Mays, M. (1996). Diagnosing latent and active pulmonary tuberculosis: A review for clinicians. *Nurse Practitioner, 21*(2), 86+.

Little, R.E. (1977). Moderate alcohol use during pregnancy and decreased infant birth weight. *American Journal of Public Health, 67,* 1154–1156.

Long, P.J. (1995). Rethinking iron supplementation during pregnancy. *Journal of Nurse-Midwifery, 40,* 36–40.

Madrigal, E. (1995, January 30). Get off my back. I have enough to carry already. *The Oregonian.*

Manning, F. (1994). Fetal biophysical assessment by ultrasound. In R. Creasy and R.K. Resnik (Eds.), *Maternal-Fetal Medicine: Principles and Practice.* Philadelphia: W.B. Saunders.

Many, A., Hill, L.M., Lazebnik, N., & Martin, J.G. (1995). The association between polyhydramnios and preterm delivery. *Obstetrics and Gynecology, 86,* 389–391.

March of Dimes. *Birth defects: Tragedy and hope.*

McFarlane, J. (1993). Abuse during pregnacy: The horror and the hope. *AWHONN'S Clinical Issues, 4*(3), 350–362.

McGregor, J.A., French, J.I., Parker, R., Draper, D., Patterson, E., Jones, W., Thorsgard, K., & McFee, J. (1995). Prevention of premature birth by screening and treatment for common genital tract infections: Results of a prospective controlled evaluation. *American Journal of Obstetrics and Gynecology, 173,* 157–167.

Medical Letter. (1995). Varicella vaccine. *The Medical Letter, 37*(951), 55–56.

Meyer, N.L., Mercer, B.M., Friedman, S.A., & Sibai, B.M. (1994). Urinary dipstick protein: A poor predictor of absent or severe proteinuria. *American Journal of Obstetrics and Gynecology, 170,* 137–141.

Mikhail, M.S., & Anyaegbunam, A. (1995). Lower urinary tract dysfunction in pregnancy: A review. (1995). *Obstetrical and Gynecological Survey, 50,* 675–683.

Moore, T.K., & Cayle, J.E. (1990). The amniotic fluid index in normal pregnancy. *American Journal of Obstetrics and Gynecology, 162,* 1168–1173.

National Academy of Sciences. (1992). *Nutrition during pregnancy and lactation: An implementation guide.* Washington, D.C.: National Academy Press.

Nelson, M.K. (1983). Working-class women, middle-class women, and models of childbirth. *Social Problems, 30,* 284–297.

Nichol, K.L., Lind, A., Margolis, K.A., Murdoch, M., McFadden, R., Hauge, M., Magnan, S., & Drake, M. (1995). The effectiveness of vaccination against influenza in healthy, working adults. *New England Journal of Medicine, 333,* 889–893.

Niebyl, J. (1995). Folic acid supplementation to prevent birth defects. *Contemporary OB/GYN, 40*(6), 43+.

Nurminen, T. (1995). Female noise exposure, shift work, and reproduction. *Journal of Occupational and Environmental Medicine, 37,* 945–950.

Office of International Health, U.S. Public Health Service. *Guidelines for analysis of sociocultural factors in health.* (1989).

Olavarrieta, C.D., & Sotelo, J. (1996). Domestic violence in Mexico. *Journal of the American Medical Association, 275*, 1937–1941.

Oregon Health Division. (1994). Hepatitis B. *Investigative Guidelines*, 1–10.

Oregon Health Division. (1995). Pelvic inflamatory disease. *CD Summary, 44*(14), 1.

Oregon Health Division. (1996a). Secondhand smoke: Another reason for parents to quit. *CD Summary, 45*(8), 1–2.

Oregon Health Division. (1996b). Medical aftermath of the Hanford Project. *CD Summary, 45*(1), 1–2.

Oregon Teen Pregnancy Task Force, Adolescent Pregnancy Prevention Subcommittee. (1966). Tough questions about adult men who have babies with babies. *Rational Enquirer*, 6.

Östgaard, H.C., Zetherstrom, G., Roos-Hansson, E., & Svanberg, B. (1994). Reduction of back and posterior pelvic pain in pregnancy. *Spine, 19*, 894–900.

Pacific Northwest Regional Genetics Group Prenatal Genetics Committee. (1995). Maternal serum multiple marker screening algorithm for practitioners. *Genetics Northwest, 10*, 4.

Perez-Stable, E.J. (1995, August 24). Infectious Diseases. Talk given at *Essentials of Primary Care: A Core Curriculum for Practice in the Managed Care Era*, Squaw Creek, North Lake Tahoe, CA. Presented by Division of Internal Medicine, University of California at San Francisco School of Medicine.

Piper, J.M., Mitchell, E.F., & Ray, W.A. (1993). Prenatal use of metronidazole and birth defects: No association. *Obstetrics and Gynecology, 82*, 348–52.

Poss, J.E., & Rangel, R. (1995). Working effectively with interpreters in the primary care setting. *Nurse Practitioner, 20*(12), 43–47.

Pritchard, J.A. (1965). Changes in the blood volume during pregnancy and delivery. *Anesthesiology, 26*, 393–399.

Public Health Service Expert Panel on the Content of Prenatal Care. (1989). *Caring for our future: The content of prenatal care.* Washington, D.C.: Department of Health and Human Services.

Randall-David, E. (1989). *Strategies for working with culturally diverse communities and clients.* Bethesda, MA: Association for the Care of Children's Health.

Redman, C., & Walker, I. (1992). *Pre-eclampsia: The facts.* New York: Oxford University Press.

Reyes, M.P., & Akhras, J. (1995). Dealing with maternal and congenital syphilis. *Contemporary OB/GYN, 40*(6), 52+.

Roberts, J.M. (1994). Pregnancy-Related Hypertension. In R. K. Creasy and R. Resnik (Eds.), *Maternal-Fetal Medicine: Principles and Practice* (3rd ed.). Philadelphia: W.B. Saunders.

Rothman, K.J., Moore, L.L., Singer, M.R., Nguyen, U.D.T., Mannino, S., & Milunsky, A. (1995). Terarogenicity of high vitamin A intake. *New England Journal of Medicine, 333*, 1369–1373.

Rouse, D.J., Andrews, W.W., Goldenberg, R.L., & Owen, J. (1995). Screening and treatment of asymptomatic bacteriuria of pregnancy to prevent pyelonephritis: A cost-effectiveness and cost-benefit analysis, *Obstetrics and Gynecology, 86*, 119–123.

Schneider, K.A. (1994). Counseling about cancer. *Genetics Northwest, 9*(1), 1–3.

Schoenfeld, A., Ziv, E., Stein, L., Zaidel, D., & Ovadia, J. (1987). Seat belts in pregnancy and the obstetrician. *Obstetrical and Gynecological Survey, 42*, 275–282.

Schneider, K. A. (1994). *Counseling about cancer: Strategies for genetic counselors.* Wallingford, PA: National Society for Genetic Counselors.

Scott, D.E. (1972). Anemia during pregnancy. *Obstetrics and Gyncology Annual, 1*, 219.

Sheon, A.R., Fox, H.E., Rick, K.C., Stratton, P., Diaz, C., Tuomala, R., Mendez, H., Carrington, J., and Alexander, G. (1996). The women and infants transmission study (WITS) of Maternal-Infant HIV transmission: Study design, methods, and baseline data. *Journal of Women's Health, 5*, 69–78.

Shulman, L.P., & Elias, S. (1993). Amniocentesis and chorionic villus sampling. *Western Journal of Medicine, 159*,

Sibai, B.M. (1996). Treatment of hypertension in pregnant women. *New England Journal of Medicine, 335*, 257–265.

Sibai, B.M., McCubbin, J.H., Anderson, G.D., Lipshitz, J., & Dilts, P.V., Jr., (1981). Eclampsia I. Observations from 67 recent cases. *Obstetrics and Gynecology, 58*, 609–.

Sickles, E. A., & Kopans, D.B. (1995). Mammographic screening for women aged 40 to 49 years: The primary care practitioner's dilemma. *Annals of Internal Medicine, 122,* 534–538.

Simkin, P. (1994). Memories that really matter. *Childbirth Educator Magazine,* 220+.

Slaughter, R., & Kanter, L. (1993). Women Being Alive. In *Domestic violence: Is it happening to you?*

Spitzer, R.L., Williams, J.B.W., Kroenke, K., Linzer, M., deGruy III, F.V., Hahn, S.R., Brody, D., & Johnson, J.G. (1994). Utility of a new procedure for diagnosing mental disorders in primary care: The PRIME-MD 1000 study. *Journal of the American Medical Association, 272,* 1749–1756.

Streissguth, A.P., Sampson, P.D., & Barr, H.B. (1989). Neurobehavioral dose-response effects of prenatal alcohol exposure in humans from infancy to adulthood. *Annals of the New York Academy of Sciences, 562,* 145–158.

Taylor, B.M. (1995). Gender-power relations and safer sex negotiation. *Journal of Advanced Nursing, 22,* 687–693.

Thompson, M.W. (1991). *Genetics in Medicine* (5th ed.). Philadelphia: W.B. Saunders.

Titus, K. (1996). When physicians ask, women tell about domestic abuse and violence. *Journal of the American Medical Association* (Medical News and Perspectives), *275,* 1863–1865.

Toglia, M.R., & DeLancey, J.O.L. (1994). Anal incontinence and the obstetrician-gynecologist. *Obstetrics and Gynecology, 84*(4, Part 2), 731–740.

Toubia, N. (1994). Female genital mutilation and the responsibility of reproductive health officials. *International Journal of Gynecology and Obstetrics. 46,* 127–135.

Turrentine, M.A., & Newton, E.R. (1995). Amoxicillin or erythromycin for the treatment of antenatal chlamydial infection: A meta-analysis. *Obstetrics and Gynecology, 86,* 1021–1025.

University of Washington School of Medicine. (1994). The Centers for Disease Control and Prevention: Sexually transmitted diseases treatment guidelines. *Clinical Courier, 12*(17), 1–7.

U.S. Department of Health and Human Services. (1989). *Caring for our future: The content of prenatal care.* Wasington, D.C.: Superintendent of Documents.

U.S. Department of Health and Human Services. (1994). *Clinician's handbook of preventive services.* Washington, D.C.: Superintendent of Documents.

U.S. Food and Drug Administration. (1993). Focus on food labeling. *FDA Consumer* (Special Report), 56–63.

U.S. Preventive Services Task Force. (1993). Routine iron supplementation during pregnancy. *Journal of the American Medical Association, 270,* 2846–2847.

Weeks, J.W., Asrat, T., Morgan, M.A., Nageotte, M., Thomas, S.J., & Freeman, R.K. (1995). Antepartum surveillance for a history of stillbirth: When should it begin? *American Journal of Obstetrics and Gynecology, 172*(2), 486–92.

Wheeler, L. (1995). Well-Woman Assessment. In C.I. Fogel & N.F. Woods (Eds.), *Women's health care: A comprehensive handbook.* Thousand Oaks, CA: Sage Publications.

Wilhelm, J., Morris, D., & Hotham, N. (1990). Epilepsy and pregnancy: A review of 98 pregnancies. *Australia and New Zealand Journal of Obstetrics and Gynecology, 4,* 290.

Williams, M V., Parker, R.M., Baker, D.W., Parikh, N.S., Pitkin, K., Coates, W.C., & Nurss, J. (1995). Inadequate functional literacy among patients at two public hospitals, *Journal of the American Medical Association, 274*(21), 1677–1682.

World Health Organization, Division of Family Health. (1994). Female genital mutilation: Prevalence and Distribution. *Female Genital Mutilation: Information Kit.* Geneva, Switzerland: World Health Organization.

Ziemer, M.M., Paone, J.P., Schupay, J., & Cole, E. (1990). Methods to prevent and manage nipple pain in breastfeeding women. *Western Journal of Nursing Research, 12,* 732–744.

Zion, A.B., & Aiman, J. (1989). Level of reading difficulty in the American College of Obstetricians and Gynecologists patient education pamphlets. *American Journal of Obstetriocs and Gynecology, 74,* 955–960.

Zuckerman, A.J. (1995). Occupational exposure to hepatitis B virus and human immunodeficiency virus: A comparative risk analysis. *American Journal of Infection Control, 23*(5), 286–289.

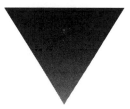

Appendices

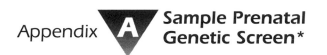

Appendix A
Sample Prenatal Genetic Screen*

Name
Patient #
Date

1. Will you be 35 years or older when the baby is due?
2. Have you, the baby's father, or anyone in either of your families ever had any of the following disorders?
   - Down syndrome (mongolism)
   - Other chromosomal abnormality
   - Neural tube defect, ie, spina bifida (meningomyelocele or open spine), anencephaly
   - Hemophilia
   - Muscular dystrophy
   - Cystic fibrosis
   If yes, indicate the relationship of the affected person to you or to the baby's father:
3. Do you or the baby's father have a birth defect?
   If yes, who has the defect and what is it?
4. In any previous marriages, have you or the baby's father had a child, born dead or alive, with a birth defect not listed in question 2 above?
   If yes, what was the defect and who had it?
5. Do you or the baby's father have any close relatives with mental retardation?
   If yes, indicate the relationship of the affected person to you or to the baby's father: Indicate the cause, if known:
6. Do you, the baby's father, or a close relative in either of your families have a birth defect, any familial disorder, or a chromosomal abnormality not listed above?
   If yes, indicate the condition and the relationship of the affected person to you or to the baby's father:
7. In any previous marriages, have you or the baby's father had a stillborn child or three or more first-trimester spontaneous pregnancy losses?
   Have either of you had a chromosomal study?
   If yes, indicate who and the results.
8. If you or the baby's father are of Jewish ancestry, have either of you been screened for Tay-Sachs disease?
   If yes, indicate who and the results.
9. If you or the baby's father are black, have either of you been screened for sickle cell trait?
   If yes, indicate who and the results.
10. If you or the baby's father are of Italian, Greek, or Mediterranean background, have either of you been tested for β-thalassemia?
    If yes, indicate who and the results.
11. If you or the baby's father are of Philippine or Southeast Asian ancestry, have either of you been tested for α-thalassemia?
    If yes, indicate who and the results.
12. Excluding iron and vitamins, have you taken any medications or recreational drugs since being pregnant or since your last menstrual period? (Include nonprescription drugs.)
    If yes, give name of medication and time taken during pregnancy.

---

*Any patient replying "YES" to questions should be offered appropriate counseling. If the patient declines further counseling or testing, this should be noted in the chart. Given that genetics is a field in a state of flux, alterations or updates to this form will be required periodically.
(Reprinted with permission from American College of Obstetricians and Gynecologists. Antenatal Diagnosis of Genetic Disorders (Technical Bulletin No. 108). Washington, D.C.: ACOG, © 1991.)

Appendix 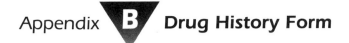 B Drug History Form

Drug	Age at First Use	How Often Used in Past Year	How Often Used This Month	Number of Times/Day When Used
Wine				
Beer				
"Hard" liquor				
Tobacco				
Marijuana				
PCP (angel dust)				
LSD				
Tranquilizers				
Heroin				
Smoking cocaine (freebasing/crack)				
Sniffing/snorting cocaine				
Skin popping				
Other cocaine				
Speedball (heroin and cocaine)				
Codeine				
Methamphetamines (crystal/speed)				
Diet pills				
Methadone				
Other (please specify)				

NOTE: The questionnaire shown here can be used to assess a woman's use of illicit drugs.

(Reprinted with permission from Wheeler, L. (1995). Well-woman assessment. In C.I. Fogel & N.F. Woods (Eds.). *Women's health care: A comprehensive handbook.* Thousand Oaks, CA: Sage Publications, p. 159.)

Appendix ▼C Environmental Exposure History Form

1. Have you ever worked at a job or hobby in which you came in contact with any of the following by breathing, touching, or ingesting (swallowing)? If yes, please check beside the name.

Acids	Chloroform	Manganese	Solvents
Alcohols	Chloroprene	Mercury	Styrene
(industrial)	Chromates	Methylene	Talc
Alkalies	Coal dust	chloride	Toluene
Ammonia	Dichlorobenzene	Nickel	TDI or MDI
Arsenic	Ethylene	PBBs	Trichloroethylene
Asbestos	dibromide	PCBs	Trinitrotoluene
Benzene	Ethylene	Perchloroethylene	Vinyl chloride
Beryllium	dichloride	Pesticides	Welding fumes
Cadmium	Fiberglass	Phenol	X rays
Carbon tetra-	Halothane	Phosgene	Other (specify)
chloride	Isocyanates	Radiation	
Chlorinated	Ketones	Rock dust	
naphthalenes	Lead	Silica powder	

2. Do you live next to or near an industrial plant, commercial business, dump site, or nonresidential property?
3. Which of the following do you have in your home? *Please circle those that apply.*

Air conditioner	Air purifier	Central heating
Gas stove	Electric stove	(gas or oil?)
Wood stove	Humidifier	Fireplace

4. Have you recently acquired new furniture or carpet, refinished furniture, or remodeled your home?
5. Have you weatherized your home recently?
6. Are pesticides or herbicides (bug or weed killers; flea and tick sprays, collars, powders, or shampoos) used in your home or garden, or on pets?
7. Do you (or any household member) have a hobby or craft?
8. Do you work on your car?
9. Have you ever changed your residence because of a health problem?
10. Does your drinking water come from a private well, city water supply, or grocery store?
11. Approximately what year was your home built?

If you answered *yes* to any of the questions, please explain.

(From Agency for Toxic Substances and Disease Registry. (1992). *Case studies in environmental medicine: Taking an exposure history.* Atlanta: U.S. Department of Health & Human Services Public Health Service.)

Appendix 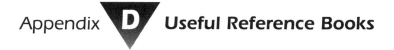 Useful Reference Books

ABUSE

Asher, A. (1994). *Please don't let him hurt me anymore.* Los Angeles: Burning Gate Press.
Bass, E., & Davis, L. (1994). *The courage to heal* (3rd ed.). New York: Harper & Row.
Doyle, R. (1996). *The woman who walked into doors.* New York: Viking.
Evans, P. (1992). *The verbally abusive relationship: How to recognize it and how to respond.* Holbrook, MA: Bob Adams.
Finney, L.D. (1992). *Reach for the rainbow: Advanced healing for survivors of sexual abuse.* New York: Putnam Publishing Group.
Foote, C. (1994). *Survivor prayers: Talking to God about childhood sexual abuse.* Louisville, KY: Westminster Press.
Graber, M.A. (1991). *Ghosts in the bedroom: A guide for partners of incest survivors.* Deerfield Beach, FL: Health Communications.
Levy, B. (1993). *Unloved and in danger: A teen's guide to breaking free of abuse.* Seattle: Seal Press.
Maltz, W. (1991). *The sexual healing journey: A guide for survivors of sexual abuse.* New York: Harper Collins.
Marecek, M. (1993). *Breaking free from partner abuse: Voices of battered women caught in the cycle of domestic violence.* Buena Park, CA: Morning Glory Press. ($7.95).
NiCarthy, G. (1986). *Getting free: A handbook for women in abusive relationships.* Seattle, WA: Seal Press.
White, E.C. (1995). *Chain chain change: For black women in abusive relationships* (3rd ed.). Seattle, WA: Seal Press. ($8.95).

ADOLESCENT PREGNANCY AND PARENTING

Dash, L. (1989). *When children want children: An inside look at the crisis of teenage parenthood.* New York: William Morrow. (Also available for $11.00 from Penguin Books.)
Lindsay, J.W. (1990). *School-age parents: The challenge of 3-generation living.* Buena Park, CA: Morning Glory Press.
Williams, C.W. (1991). *Black teenage mothers: Pregnancy and childrearing from their perspective.* Lexington, MA: Lexington Books.

ADOPTION

Arms, S. (1990). A handful of hope. Berkeley: Celestial Arts.
Brodzinsky, D.M., Schechter, M.D., & Henig, R.M. (1992). Adoption: The lifelong search for self. New York: Doubleday.
Krementz, J. (1988). How it feels to be adopted. New York: Alfred P. Knopf.
Melina, L.R. (1989). Making sense of adoption. New York: Harper & Row.

BREASTFEEDING

Lawrence, R. (1994). *Breastfeeding: A guide for the medical profession.* St. Louis: Mosby.
Jolley, S. (1996). The breastfeeding triage tool. Seattle, WA: Seattle–King County Department of Public Health. $10. Phone: 206-296-4672; Fax: 206-296-46790.

HOMELESS WOMEN

Nietzke, A. (1994). *Natalie on the street*. Corvallis, OR: Calyx Books.
Hirsch, K. (1989). *Songs from the alley*. New York: Ticknor & Fields.
Liebow, E. (1993). *Tell them who I am: The lives of homeless women*. New York: Free Press.

NUTRITION

Institute of Medicine. (1992). *Nutrition during pregnancy and lactation: An implementation guide*. Washington, D.C.: National Academy Press. (Approximately $13.00).

PARENTING

Glenn, S. Developing Capable People. A set of six audiocassette tapes, $49.95, from Empowering People, Box B, Provo, UT, 84603, 1-800-456-7770.
Nelsen, J. (1987). *Positive discipline*. New York: Ballantine Books.
Merritt, J. (1992). *Empowering children*. Portland, OR: Parenting Resources. Available for $8.95 from 2803 S.W. Hume Court, Portland, OR, 97219.

PERINATAL LOSS

Ilse, Sherokee. (1990). *Empty arms*. Available for about $7.50 from ICEA, Box 20048, Minneapolis, MN, 55420; 1-800-624-4934; Fax: 1-612-854-8772.

POSTPARTUM DEPRESSION

Kendall-Tackett, K.A., & Kantor, G.K. (1993). *Postpartum depression: A comprehensive approach for nurses*. Newbury Park, CA: Sage. (About $16.00).
Pacific Post Partum Support Society. (1994). *Post partum depression and anxiety: A self-help guide for mothers*. (3rd ed.). Vancouver: Pacific Postpartum Support Society. (About $12.00). Order from Pacific Postpartum Support Society, 1416 Commercial Dr., #104, Vancouver, B.C. V5L 3X9 Canada.

PREPARATION FOR CHILDBIRTH

Lieberman, A.B. (1992). *Easing labor pain: The complete guide to a more comfortable and rewarding birth*. Boston: Harvard Common Press.
Odent, M. (1992). *The nature of birth and breastfeeding*. Westport, CT: Bergin & Garvey.

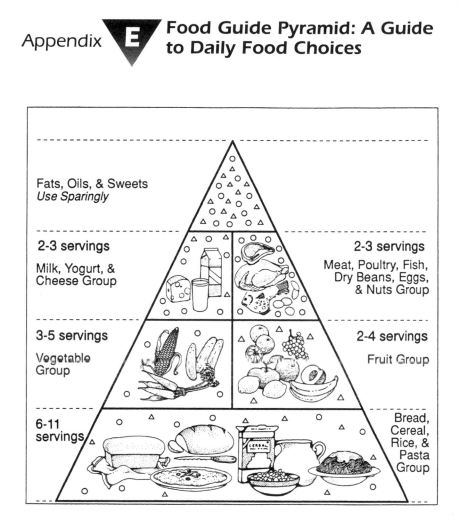

Fats, Oils, & Sweets
Use Sparingly

2-3 servings

Milk, Yogurt, & Cheese Group

2-3 servings

Meat, Poultry, Fish, Dry Beans, Eggs, & Nuts Group

3-5 servings

Vegetable Group

2-4 servings

Fruit Group

6-11 servings

Bread, Cereal, Rice, & Pasta Group

GETTING SPECIFIC

Here are examples and meanings of descriptive words for specific nutrients:

Sugar

Sugar free: less than 0.5 grams (g) per serving
No added sugar, Without added sugar, No sugar added:
- No sugars added during processing or packing, including ingredients that contain sugars (for example, fruit juices, applesauce, or dried fruit).
- Processing does not increase the sugar content above the amount naturally present in the ingredients. (A functionally insignificant increase in sugars is acceptable from processes used for purposes other than increasing sugar content.)
- The food that it resembles and for which it substitutes normally contains added sugars.
- If the food doesn't meet the requirements for a low- or reduced-calorie food, the product bears a statement that the food is not low-calorie or calorie-reduced and directs consumers' attention to the nutrition panel for further information on sugars and calorie content.

Reduced sugar: at least 25 percent less sugar per serving than reference food

Calories

Calorie free: fewer than 5 calories per serving
Low calorie: 40 calories or less per serving and if the serving is 30 g or less or 2 tablespoons or less, per 50 g of the food
Reduced or Fewer calories: at least 25 percent fewer calories per serving than reference food

Fat

Fat free: less than 0.5 g of fat per serving
Saturated fat free: less than 0.5 g per serving and the level of trans fatty acids does not exceed 1 percent of total fat
Low fat: 3 g or less per serving, and if the serving is 30 g or less or 2 tablespoons or less, per 50 g of the food
Low saturated fat: 1 g or less per serving and not more than 15 percent of calories from saturated fatty acids
Reduced or less fat: at least 25 percent less per serving than reference food
Reduced or Less saturated fat: at least 25 percent less per serving than reference food

Cholesterol

Cholesterol free: less than 2 milligrams (mg) of cholesterol and 2 g or less of saturated fat per serving
Low cholesterol: 20 mg or less and 2 g or less of saturated fat per serving and, if the serving is 30 g or less or 2 tablespoons or less, per 50 g of the food
Reduced or Less cholesterol: at least 25 percent less and 2 g or less of saturated fat per serving than reference food

Sodium

Sodium free: less than 5 mg per serving
Low sodium: 140 mg or less per serving and, if the serving is 30 g or less or 2 tablespoons or less, per 50 g of the food
Very low sodium: 35 mg or less per serving and, if the serving is 30 g or less or 2 tablespoons or less, per 50 g of the food
Reduced or Less sodium: at least 25 percent less per serving than reference food

Fiber

High fiber: 5 g or more per serving. (Foods making high-fiber claims must meet the definition for low fat, or the level of total fat must appear next to the high-fiber claim.)
Good source of fiber: 2.5 g to 4.9 g per serving
More or Added fiber: at least 2.5 g more per serving than reference food

KEY ASPECTS OF THE NEW NUTRITION LABEL

A number of consumer studies conducted by FDA, as well as outside groups, enabled FDA and the Food Safety and Inspection Service of the U.S. Department of Agriculture to agree on a new nutrition label. The new label is seen as offering the best opportunity to help consumers make informed food choices and to understand how a particular food fits into the total daily diet.

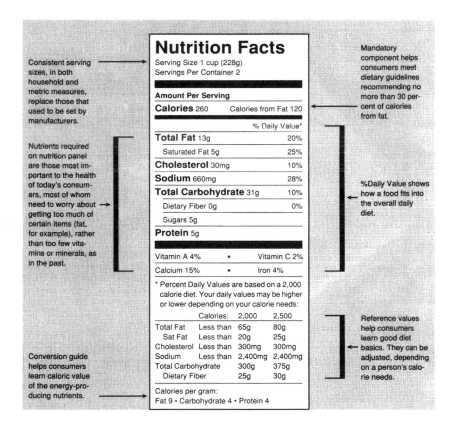

HOW TO USE THE DAILY FOOD GUIDE

What Counts As One Serving?

BREADS, CEREALS, RICE, AND PASTA
1 slice of bread
½ cup of cooked rice or pasta
½ cup of cooked cereal
1 ounce of ready-to-eat cereal

VEGETABLES
½ cup of chopped raw or cooked vegetables
1 cup of leafy raw vegetables

FRUITS
1 piece of fruit or melon wedge
¾ cup of juice
½ cup of canned fruit
¼ cup of dried fruit

MILK, YOGURT, AND CHEESE
1 cup of milk or yogurt
1½ to 2 ounces of cheese

MEAT, POULTRY, FISH, DRY BEANS, EGGS, AND NUTS
2½ to 3 ounces of cooked lean meat, poultry, or fish
Count ½ cup of cooked beans, or 1 egg, or 2 tablespoons of peanut butter as 1 ounce of lean meat (about ⅓ serving)

FATS, OILS, AND SWEETS
LIMIT CALORIES FROM THESE especially if you need to lose weight

---

The amount you eat may be more than one serving. For example, a dinner portion of spaghetti would count as two or three servings of pasta.

How Many Servings Do You Need Each Day?

Calorie level*	about 1,600	about 2,200	about 2,800
Bread group	6	9	11
Vegetable group	3	4	5
Fruit group	2	3	4
Milk group	**2–3	**2–3	**2–3
Meat group	2, for a total of 5 ounces	2, for a total of 6 ounces	3, for a total of 7 ounces

---

* These are the calorie levels if you choose lowfat, lean foods from the 5 major food groups and use foods from the fats, oils, and sweets group sparingly.

** Women who are pregnant or breastfeeding, teenagers, and young adults to age 24 need 3 servings.

A Closer Look at Fat and Added Sugars

The small tip of the Pyramid shows fats, oils, and sweets. These are foods such as salad dressings, cream, butter, margarine, sugars, soft drinks, candies, and sweet desserts. Alcoholic beverages are also part of this group. These foods provide calories but few vitamins and minerals. Most people should go easy on foods from this group.

Some fat or sugar symbols are shown in the other food groups. That's to remind you that some foods in these groups can also be high in fat and added sugars, such as cheese or ice cream from the milk group, or french fries from the vegetable group. When choosing foods for a healthful diet, consider the fat and added sugars in your choices from all the food groups, not just fats, oils, and sweets from the Pyramid tip.

Source: US Department of Agriculture/US Department of Health and Human Services

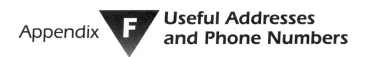
ABUSE

Incest Survivors Anonymous (ISA)
Box 5613
Long Beach, CA 90805

National Council on Child Abuse and Family Violence
1-800-222-2000

National Coalition Against Domestic Violence
1-800-333-SAFE
202-293-8860

National Council on Child Abuse and Family Violence
1155 Connecticut Ave. NW
Washington, D.C. 20036
1-800-222-2000/202-429-6695

V.O.I.C.E.S. (Victims of Incest Can Emerge Survivors)
312-327-1500

ADOPTION

International Soundex Reunion Registry (for people looking for a birth parent or
    wanting to be found; enclose a self-addressed, stamped envelope)
Box 2312
Carson City, Nevada 89702
702-882-7755

National Adoption Information Clearinghouse
11426 Rockville Pike, Suite 410
Rockville, MD 20852

Old Friends Information Services
1 Camino Sobrante, #21
Orinda, CA 94563
510-254-3646

This group does not do adoption searches, but does try to locate people who have
been known to the searcher in the past. The initial fee is $70. If the person sought
agrees to contact, there is another $50 fee.

AIDS

AIDS Clinical Trials Information Service
1-800-TRIALS-A

National AIDS Hotline
English (24 hours a day): 1-800-342-2437
Spanish (5 am–11 pm): 1-800-344-7432
TTY service for the deaf (7 am–7 pm weekdays): 1-800-243-7889

National AIDS Information Clearinghouse
1-800-458-5231

ALCOHOL AND DRUGS

Al-Anon
1-800-344-2666

American Council on Alcoholism
1-800-527-5344

800 Cocaine (Has lists of treatment centers and
support groups throughout the country)
1-800-262-2463

National Clearinghouse on Alcohol and Drug Information (NCADI)
1-800-729-6686

National Council on Alcohol and Drug Dependency
1-800-622-2255

National Council on Alcoholism
1-800-622-2255

National Drug and Alcohol Treatment Information
1-800-622-HELP

CANCER

American Cancer Society
1-800-ACS-2345

Cancer Information Service
1-800-4-CANCER

Susan G. Komer Breast Cancer Foundation
Occidental Tower
500 LBJ Freeway, Suite 370
Dallas, TX 75244
214-450-1777
Fax: 214-450-1710
Help Line: 1-800-462-9273

DEPRESSION

National Foundation for Depressive Illness
Box 2257
New York, NY 10116
1-800-248-4344

A recorded message describes the symptoms of depression and manic depression and gives the above address to write for more information, including a list of treatment centers. Requested donation is $5 but also available free. Request must include a self-addressed envelope with stamps totaling $1.01.

National Mental Health Association
1021 Prince St.
Alexandria, VA 23314-2971
1-800-969-6642

EATING DISORDERS

Eating Disorders Helpline
1-800-382-2832

National Association of Anorexia Nervosa and Associated Disorders
708-831-3438

ENVIRONMENTAL EXPOSURE

CARE Northwest (Counseling and Advice on Reproductive Exposures)
1-800-859-5343

Enviro-Health
1-800-643-4794

Part of the National Institute of Environmental Health Sciences. They perform on-line computer searches over the phone or in-depth research on environmental exposures and individual susceptibility.

MotherRisk Program
416-813-6780

Counseling about the safety of exposure to drugs, chemicals, or radiation during pregnancy or breast-feeding from specialists at the Hospital for Sick Children in Toronto, Canada.

National Medical Service
2300 Stratford Ave.
Willow Grove, PA 19090

Women with silicone breast implants can have their breast milk tested for the presence of silicone by sending 4 cc's of fresh breast milk at room temperature in a plastic container to the above company. The sample should be sent by overnight mail on a Monday or a Thursday as the test is only run on Tuesday and Friday. The lab code is #4190.

National Pesticide Telecommunications Network
1-800-858-7378

Information from the Environmental Protection Agency about the toxicity of specific pesticides.

GENETICS

Alliance of Genetic Support Groups
1-800-336-GENE

National Organization for Rare Disorders
1-800-999-6673

HOMOSEXUALITY

National Gay and Lesbian Crisis Hotline
1-800-221-7044
212-529-1604

National Lesbian and Gay Health Association
1407 S St., NW
Washington, D.C. 20009
202-939-7880

Federation of Parents and Friends of Lesbians and Gays (P-FLAG)
1101 14th St., NW
Suite 1030
Washington, D.C.
202-638-4200

INCONTINENCE

Simon Foundation for Incontinence
1-800-23-SIMON

LABOR SUPPORT

Doulas of North America (DONA)
Fax: 206-325-0472

LOSS

Compassionate Friends
Box 3696
Oak Brook, IL 60522-3696

NUTRITION

Institute of Medicine. (1992). *Nutrition during pregnancy and lactation: An implementation guide.* Washington, D.C.: National Academy Press. (Approximately $13.00).

POSTPARTUM DEPRESSION

Depression after Delivery
1-800-944-4773

Pacific Post Partum Support Society
1416 Commercial Drive, Suite 104
Vancouver, BC Canada V5L 3X9

SEXUALLY TRANSMITTED DISEASES

American Social Health Association (a nonprofit organization dedicated to stopping STDs). Operates informational hotlines 24 hours a day and publishes free brochures: 1-800-972-8500

National Herpes Hotline (operated by the American Social Health Association, 6 am–4 pm weekdays): 1-919-361-8488

STD Hot Line (operated by CDC, 5 am–8 pm weekdays): 1-800-227-8922

OTHER

Centers for Disease Control and Prevention (CDC)
404-639-3311

Down Syndrome Society
1-800-221-4602

Institute of Medicine
202-334-2169

National Academy of Sciences
202-334-2000

National Institutes of Health
301-496-4000

Sickle Cell Disease Association of America
1-800-421-8453

SIDS Alliance
1-800-221-SIDS

Spina Bifida Association of America
1-800-621-3141

Appendix G ▼ Prime-MD Tool to Screen for Mental Disorders

PATIENT QUESTIONNAIRE

Name: Age:

Sex: Male   Female   Today's Date:

INSTRUCTIONS: This questionnaire will help in understanding problems that you may have. It may be necessary to ask you more questions about some of these items. Please make sure to check a box for *every* item.

During the PAST MONTH, have you been bothered A LOT by . . .

1. stomach pain
2. back pain
3. pain in your arms, legs, or joints (knees, hips, etc)
4. menstrual pain or problems
5. pain or problems during sexual intercourse
6. headaches
7. chest pain
8. dizziness
9. fainting spells
10. feeling your heart pound or race
11. shortness of breath
12. constipation, loose bowels, or diarrhea
13. nausea, gas, or indigestion
14. feeling tired or having low energy
15. trouble sleeping
16. your eating being out of control
17. little interest or pleasure in doing things
18. feeling down, depressed, or hopeless
19. "nerves" or feeling anxious or on edge
20. worrying about a lot of different things

During the PAST MONTH . . .

21. have you had an anxiety attack (suddenly feeling fear or panic)
22. have you thought you should cut down on your drinking of alcohol
23. has anyone complained about your drinking
24. have you felt guilty or upset about your drinking
25. was there ever a single day in which you had five or more drinks of beer, wine, or liquor

Overall, would you say your health is:

Excellent
Very good
Good
Fair
Poor

_____
Updated for DSM-IV™

Appendix H

Responses to a Disclosure of Childhood Sexual Abuse

1. Invite disclosure. Ask appropriate questions and let the survivor know that you are willing to discuss whatever she feels comfortable telling you about her past. Let her set the limits regarding details; if you push details, do so gently.
2. Comment on her courage. It is often very difficult to talk about past abuse and long-held secrets. She was courageous to have survived her past and she is courageous to discuss it now with you. Let her know that you are sorry that she had to go through such things.
3. Try to be calm and matter-of-fact. She does not need a highly emotional response, but she does need accepting, encouraging support.
4. A child is *never* to blame for the abuse, no matter what the circumstances. Emphasize that for her, and be careful of questions that sound blaming. ("Did you tell anyone?")
5. Believe her. Don't try to deny what happened. Survivors can be experts of minimizing or denial. Gently let her know that you think what happened is important, and that you will not participate in her denial. She is a valuable person, and whatever happened to her was not "OK," or "Not so bad."
6. Take time to listen. Don't try to rush her. It may take a long time for her to disclose the details of her abuse. This may happen slowly over many appointments. Respect her ability to set the pace, no matter how long it takes.
7. Have faith in her ability to heal. She really does not know what is her best path to healing, but she may need your help and support in identifying her needs. Ask "Do you know what would help you?" Ask for permission before you offer a hug or a touch.
8. Become an expert in referral. Know the resources in your area and encourage her to seek therapy if she has not already done so. Groups can be especially helpful for survivors. Remember you are not a therapist, but you can be a sensitive support person. Offer her hope.
9. Respect her confidentiality. Never discuss her disclosure with anyone without her permission. Let her know what you are writing in her chart and why. If she leads you to believe there are other children still at risk for abuse, you are obligated to report this. Discuss with her the necessity of reporting, but do so gently with lots of support.
10. Check in with her periodically to find out how she is doing, what support she might need, and what else is coming up. If she does not want to talk about it, respect that, but don't let the dialogue stop because you are not open to it.
11. Do your own healing work. Your support will come from a stronger place if you have dealt with your own feelings.

(By Christine Heritage, CNM, Cottage Grove, OR. Reprinted with permission.)

Appendix ▼I Guidelines for Working With an Interpreter

1. Meet regularly with the interpreter to keep communications open and facilitate an understanding of the goals and purpose of the interview or counseling session. Certainly you should meet with the interpreter before meeting with the client.
2. Encourage the interpreter to meet with the client before the interview to find out about the client's educational level and attitudes toward health and health care. This information can aid the interpreter in the depth and type of information and explanation that will be needed.
3. Speak in short units of speech—not long, involved sentences or paragraphs. Avoid long, complex discussions of several topics in a single interview.
4. Avoid technical terminology, abbreviations, and professional jargon.
5. Avoid colloquialisms, abstractions, idiomatic expressions, slang, similes, and metaphors.
6. Encourage the interpreter to translate the client's own words as much as possible rather than paraphrasing or "polishing" it into professional jargon. This gives a better sense of the client's concept of what is going on, his or her emotional state, and other important information.
7. Encourage the interpreter to refrain from inserting his or her own ideas or interpretations, or omitting information.
8. To check on the client's understanding and the accuracy of the translation, ask the client to repeat instructions or whatever has been communicated in his or her own words, with the translator facilitating.
9. During the interaction, look at and speak directly to the client, not the interpreter.
10. Listen to the client and watch his or her nonverbal communication. Often you can learn a lot regarding the affective aspects of the client's response by observing facial expressions, voice intonations, and body movements.
11. Be patient. An interpreted interview takes longer. Careful interpretation often requires that the interpreter use long explanatory phrases.

Even if you are using an interpreter, there are ways you can become more actively involved in the communication process.

1. Learn proper forms of address in the client's language. Use of these titles conveys respect for the client and demonstrates your willingness to learn about his or her culture.
2. Learn basic words and sentences of the client's language. Become familiar with special terminology used by clients. Even though you can't speak well enough to communicate directly, the more you understand, the greater the chance you will pick up on misinterpretations and misunderstandings in the interpreter–client interchange.
3. Use a positive tone of voice that conveys your interest in the client. Never be condescending, judgmental, or patronizing.
4. Repeat important information more than once. Always give the reason or purpose for a treatment or prescription.
5. Reinforce verbal interaction with materials written in the client's language and with visual aids.

NONVERBAL COMMUNICATION

Much of what is communicated is not verbalized but conveyed through facial expressions and body movements that are specific to each culture. It is important to understand the cross-cultural variations in order to avoid misunderstandings and unintentional offenses.

Silence. Some cultures are quite comfortable with long periods of silence while others consider it appropriate to speak before the other person has finished talking. Learn about the appropriate use of pauses or interruptions in your client's culture.

Distance. Some cultures are comfortable with close body space, while others are more comfortable at greater distance. In general, Anglo Americans prefer to be about an arm's length away from another person while Hispanics prefer closer proximity and Asians prefer greater distance. Give your client the choice by inviting him or her to "have a seat wherever you like."

Eye contact. Some cultures advise their members to look people straight in the eye (Anglos) while others consider it disrespectful (blacks), a sign of hostility or impoliteness (Asians, Native Americans). Observe the client when talking and listening to get cues regarding appropriate eye contact.

(From Randall-David, E. (1989). *Strategies for working with culturally diverse communities and clients*, pp. 32–33.) Reproduced with permission of The Association for the Care of Children's Health, 7910 Woodmont Ave., Suite 300, Bethesda, MD 20814.

Appendix J

Agents Associated With Adverse Female Reproductive Capacity or Developmental Effects in Human and Animal Studies*

Agent	Human Outcomes	Strength of Association in Humans[†]	Animal Outcomes	Strength of Association in Animals[†]
Anesthetic gases**	Reduced fertility, spontaneous abortion	1, 3	Birth defects	1,3
Arsenic	Spontaneous abortion, low birth weight	1	Birth defects, fetal loss	2
Benzo(a)pyrene	None	NA[§]	Birth defects	1
Cadmium	None	NA	Fetal loss, birth defects	2
Carbon disulfide	Menstrual disorders, spontaneous abortion	1	Birth defects	1
Carbon monoxide	Low birth weight, fetal death (high doses)	1	Birth defects, neonatal mortality	2
Chlordecone	None	NA	Fetal loss	2, 3
Chloroform	None	NA	Fetal loss	1
Chloroprene	None	NA	Birth defects	2, 3
Ethylene glycol ethers	Spontaneous abortion	1	Birth defects	2
Ethylene oxide	Spontaneous abortion	1	Fetal loss	1
Formamides	None	NA	Fetal loss, birth defects	2
Inorganic mercury**	Menstrual disorders, spontaneous abortion	1	Fetal loss, birth defects	1
Lead**	Spontaneous abortion, prematurity, neurologic dysfunction in child	2	Birth defects, fetal loss	2
Organic mercury	CNS malformation, cerebral palsy	2	Birth defects, fetal loss	2
Physical stress	Prematurity	2	None	NA
Polybrominated biphenyls (PBBs)	None	NA	Fetal loss	2
Polychlorinated biphenyls (PCBs)	Neonatal PCB syndrome (low birth weight, hyperpigmentation, eye abnormalities)	2	Low birth weight, fetal loss	2
Radiation, ionizing	Menstrual disorders, CNS defects, skeletal & eye anomalies, mental retardation, childhood cancer	2	Fetal loss, birth defects	2
Selenium	Spontaneous abortion	3	Low birth weight, birth defects	2
Tellurium	None	NA	Birth defects	2
2,4-Dichlorophenoxyacetic acid (2,4-D)	Skeletal defects	4	Birth defects	1
2,4,5-Trichlorophenoxyacetic acid (2,4,5-T)	Skeletal defects	4	Birth defects	1
Video display terminals	Spontaneous abortion	4	Birth defects	1
Vinyl chloride**	CNS defects	1	Birth defects	1, 4
Xylene	Menstrual disorders, fetal loss	1	Fetal loss, birth defects	1

* Major studies of the reproductive health effects of exposure to dioxin are currently in progress.

[†] 1 = limited positive data.   3 = limited negative data.
   2 = strong positive data.   4 = strong negative data.

[§] Not applicable because no adverse outcomes were observed.

** Symbol used to designate agents that may have male-mediated effects.

(From *Case studies in environmental studies: Reproductive and developmental hazards.* (1993). Washington, D.C.: Department of Health and Human Services, p. 4.)

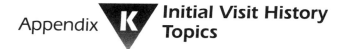

Appendix **K** Initial Visit History Topics

MENSTRUAL HISTORY/DATING

LMP, including cycle frequency and length of most recent menses
Pregnancy test (date)
Quickening

CONTRACEPTIVE HISTORY

Ever-used methods and reasons for stopping
Most recently used method and last use

OB HISTORY

TPAL
Type of delivery
Length of gestation
Length of labor
Birth weight
Gender
Complications including congenital anomalies
Current health of children and where they are living
Feelings about previous pregnancy or birth experiences, including use of analgesia or
    anesthesia

MED-SURG HISTORY (not essential)

GYN problems including HPV, herpes, gonorrhea, chlamydia, syphilis, PID, abnormal
    Pap and date of last Pap
Organic disease
Surgery, accidents, ER visits, hospitalizations, including blood products between 1978
    and 1985
Psychiatric problems, including diagnosed mental illness, depression, anxiety, mania,
    panic attacks, eating disorders
Foreign travel or residence
Sexual history, including problems, multiple partners/safe sex practices, age at first
    coitus
Abuse (physical, emotional, sexual)
Nontraditional healing practices
Medications (current and past), including over-the-counter, prescription, herbal reme-
    dies, potential teratogens, allergies

FAMILY HISTORY

Risk for genetic disease, including ethnic background
Organic disease
Psychiatric illness
Observing family violence
Abuse of alcohol or drugs
Father of baby's family, including ethnic background, three or more miscarriages, stillbirth, mental retardation, birth defect, genetic or chromosome abnormality, blood
Obstetrical history, including three or more miscarriages, fraternal twins in the maternal line, DES in mother, severe preeclampsia in mother or sisters
Feelings if adopted
Father's use/abuse of alcohol or drugs
Consanguinity

ENVIRONMENTAL EXPOSURES, INCLUDING TOXIC AGENTS AND X-RAYS

HABITS UNDERMINING HEALTH (SMOKING, ALCOHOL, DRUGS)

SOCIAL HISTORY

Place of birth
Family constellation and status of relationships (FOB, children, parents, sibs)
Living situation: frequency of moving, kind of dwelling, number of people, safety, food
Occupation including financial circumstances, lifting or standing, change of shifts
Education (highest grade completed, literacy)
Hobbies, interests, and goals
Religious preference
Pets
Foreign travel
Sources of support
Sources of stress

HEALTH HABITS

Safety: seat belts, smoke alarms, weapons
Exercise
Breast and skin exams
Immunizations
Nutritional practices/supplements
Nontraditional healers/health practices

Appendix L

Sample Initial Prenatal Visit Charting of Historical Information

Donna is an 18-year-old gravida 1 who comes for her first prenatal visit accompanied by BF/FOB, Brian, age 23. This pregnancy is unplanned but accepted, and Donna intends to raise the baby with help from her mother.

MENSTRUAL HISTORY

LMP/LNMP: March 7, regular cycles every 28–30 days

CONTRACEPTIVE HISTORY

Oral contraceptives ×6 mos at age 15, occ condoms since then, no condoms in last 6 mos

OB HISTORY: NA

MED-SURG HISTORY

UTI 2 years ago
Thinks she needs glasses—never tested
No chickenpox

GYN History: Neg
Sexual Problems: 0

MEDS

Amoxicillin 2 years ago for UTI
Occ Tylenol before pregnancy

Prenatal vitamins for last 2 weeks
No allergies

PETS: None

FAMILY HISTORY

Mother born in Nebraska, father born in Maine
Medical hx: PGF was alcoholic, died in car accident
Drug abuse: father is alcoholic
Relationships: parents divorced when Donna was 6 years old
Ethnic background: Euro-American
Severe preeclampsia: 0

ENVIRONMENTAL EXPOSURES: None known

FOREIGN TRAVEL: None

HEALTH HABITS

Sleep: OK
Safety: Uses seat belts; 2 smoke alarms—batteries recently changed, no weapons at
home
Health-promoting habits:
No regular exercise program
Does not do SBE or monthly skin check
Does not use sunscreen
Usual childhood immunizations, no recent TD, no Hep B, no PPD, no HIV testing
No recent dental or vision check
Never diets
Total of 3 sexual partners, monogamous at present, sporadic use of condoms, initial
sexual experience at age 16
Nontraditional health practices/practitioners: 0
Nutrition: low in fruits and veggies, good protein and fiber, moderate fat
Habits undermining health:
Cigarettes: 0
Alcohol: 0
Illicit drugs: Never

SOCIAL HISTORY

Place of birth: Oregon, infrequent moves
Relationships: BF/FOB, Brian, is unemployed and lives with an older brother. He reports that parents were heavy drug users when he was in school, says he was phys-
ically and emotionally abused; denies sexual abuse; rates relationship with him a 6
Other relationships: Mother is teacher's aide. Rates relationship with mother a 7 on a
scale of 1 to 10. Rates relationship with sibs an 8. Mother is supportive but involved
with new boyfriend; father lives in Florida, phones occasionally, Donna does not
miss him.
Religious preference: None
Living situation: Lives with mother and 6- and 10-year-old brothers in 3 BR apt. In safe
area.
Occupation: Works about 30 hours per week at Burger King, may stand 4 hours at a
time; likes job
Education: Quit school in 11th grade, was not doing well
Goals: Thinks she would like to be an x-ray technician
Hobbies/interests: Singing and dancing
Abuse: 0
Finances: "Tight," on Oregon Health Plan and WIC
Sources of support: Mother, maternal aunt who lives nearby, 2 best friends, Brian at
times
Major stressors: (1) Conflict with Brian about his not working and (2) His heavy use of
marijuana.

THIS PREGNANCY

Dating
Preg test: pos urine at Planned Parenthood April 13
Quickening: July 15
Vomiting daily in first trimester
Continuing breast tenderness
No pica

Chart for Estimating Body Mass Index (BMI)

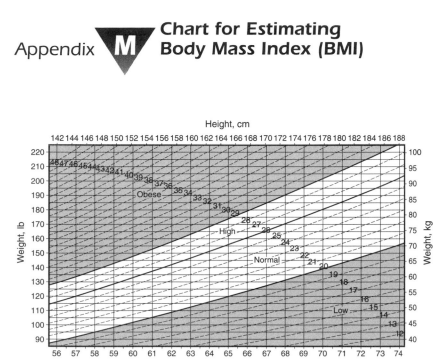

Appendix N

Female Circumcision and Map Demonstrating Where It Is Practiced

An estimated two million girls are at risk for female circumcision each year (World Health Organization, 1994). In Africa, the procedure is usually carried out on young, preadolescent, or adolescent girls by an older village woman as part of a traditional village rite that ensures that girls are marriageable. Varying amounts of clitoral and labial tissue are removed, often with a razor blade, scissors, knife, or sharpened stone. In one type of circumcision, partial or total amputation of the clitoris occurs. In these situations intercourse and labor occur without obstruction. In some instances, the upper ⅔ of the labia majora are also removed, leaving an opening over the urethra and vagina. The most extensive form of female circumcision, also known as infibulation or pharaonic circumcision, involves removal of the clitoris and the labia minora, plus an incision of the labia majora to create raw surfaces which are either stitched or approximated with thorns so that the urethra and the vagina are covered. A small opening is left so that urine and menstrual blood can pass through. The infibulation may be cut at first intercourse.

The type of procedure performed may not be apparent upon inspection of the genitalia, as the amount of cutting varies from one operator to another and complications can influence the appearance of the scar. Movement by the child, the amount of light available for visualization, and the tool used for the incisions will influence the extent of cutting. Complications include hemorrhage, local and systemic infection, urinary retention, incontinence, scarring, sexual dysfunction, lifelong pain, chronic pelvic infections, vesicovaginal and recto-vaginal fistulas, infertility, gangrene, tetanus, shock, septicemia, and death.

The most common complication is the formation of dermoid cysts in the line of the scar, as a result of embedded epithelial cells and sebaceous glands in the stitched area. Dermoid cysts as small as a pea or as large as a football have been reported. Keloid formation is another disfiguring complication, which, together with dermoid cysts, causes much anxiety, shame, and fear in women who think that their genitalia are re-growing in monstrous shapes or fear they may have cancer. A painful stitch neuroma may develop as a result of a nerve ending being trapped in the scar. This can cause severe dyspareunia, which may prohibit intercourse. Recurrent stitch abscesses and splitting of poorly healed scars, particularly over the area of the clitoral artery, can plague the woman and her physician for many years (Toubia, p. 130-131).

Unsterile instruments and the likelihood of tearing the small vaginal opening with intercourse increase the risk for HIV transmission. The psychological and sexual effects of female circumcision have not been studied.

214

AREAS OF THE WORLD WHERE FEMALE
CIRCUMCISION IS FOUND

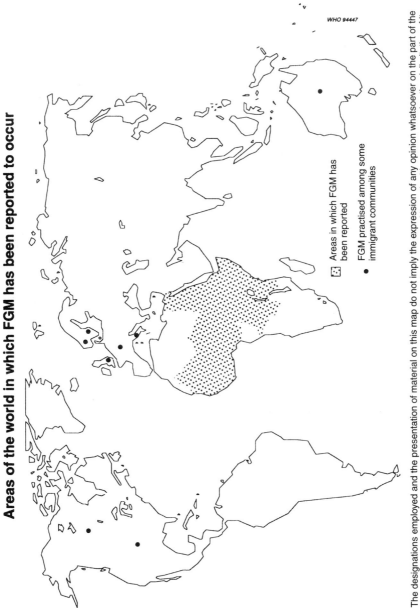

Areas of the world in which FGM has been reported to occur

WHO 94447

Areas in which FGM has been reported

FGM practised among some immigrant communities

The designations employed and the presentation of material on this map do not imply the expression of any opinion whatsoever on the part of the World Health Organization concerning the legal status of any country, territory, city or area or of its authorities, or concerning the delimitation of its frontiers or boundaries. Information on the map is based mainly on partial and incomplete data.

Appendix ▽ Criteria for Determining a Positive Tuberculosis Skin Test

1. Read in 48 to 72 hours but positive reactions may still be measurable up to 1 week after testing
2. Classification as positive
   a. 5 mm or more
      (1) Close, recent contact
      (2) X-ray, suggesting old, healed lesion
      (3) Known or suspected HIV infection
   b. 10 mm or more
      (1) Risk factors known to increase tbc risk
      (2) Foreign-born, from high prevalence area (Asia, Africa, Latin America)
      (3) Medically underserved, low-income, especially African American, Hispanic, and Native American
      (4) IV drug user

Appendix P

Summary of Clinician Activities to Prepare for the Return Prenatal Visit

1. Write down thoughts about additional information to gather as the client's record is reviewed.
2. Note demographic information and any social history available.
3. Review the obstetric data.
4. Review the medical history.
5. Review the family history.
6. Review initial physical examination findings.
7. Review all laboratory results.
8. Review dating data and conclusions.
9. If client is a smoker, note interest in cutting down or quitting. If interested, note plans, including any involvement in a smoking-cessation program.
10. Note the BMI and recommended weight gain.
11. Review the problem list.
12. Review record for previously noted concerns/complaints/discomforts and any treatment recommended.
13. Review form titled "Important Data and Key Moments" and correlate the gestational age of the client's baby with the suggested activities.
14. Note data available at today's visit:
    Blood pressure
    Results of urine testing
    Weight (noting total gain to date and gain since last visit)

Appendix ▼Q Antepartum Revisit Form for Patients to Complete

PRENATAL REVISIT QUESTIONS

Since your last visit have you had:
Headaches
Problems with your eyes (blurred vision, blind spots, flashing lights or lines)
Swelling of your
  face
  hands
  legs
  feet
Pain in your
  chest
  back
  legs
  abdomen
Problems with urination (peeing) such as
  burning
  leaking urine
  not being able to wait to use the toilet
  pain
Bleeding or spotting from your vagina (birth canal)
Leaking fluid from your vagina (water from the bag of waters)
Vaginal discharge
  burning
  itching
  change in the discharge
  bad smell to discharge
  increase in amount
Sores or growths in the genital area (private parts)
Illnesses or fever
Exposure to children or adults who were sick with an infection
Skin rashes or itching
Signs of labor such as
  contractions
  cramping
  pelvic pressure
  low backache
Accidents or falls OR being hit, pushed, shoved, beaten by someone (even if it was just one time)
Changes in the way the baby moves
Craving anything to eat or to smell
Visits to another doctor, nurse, clinic, emergency room or hospital

Since your last visit, write down:
Any medicines you have used (prescription or over-the-counter)
Any plants or herbs/herbal teas you have used to help you feel better or treat an illness
Any street or illegal drugs you have used
The kind and amount of alcohol you have used
The number of cigarettes you have smoked per day
Since your last visit, have you been hit, hurt, or threatened?
Do you need any prenatal vitamins; iron tablets; any other medicines?

There are many common discomforts of pregnancy. If there is a particular one that is bothering you or that you want information about, or help or suggestions for how to work with or relieve the discomfort, please mark below. If none of these worry or bother you, skip this section.

Nausea (feeling sick to your stomach)	Vomiting (throwing up)
Diarrhea	Constipation
Hemorrhoids	Not feeling hungry
Heartburn	Breast tenderness
Varicose veins	Trouble sleeping
Shortness of breath	Numbness or tingling of hands or legs or feet
Tired all the time (fatigue)	Leg cramps
Sciatica (sharp pains down your leg)	Backache
Heart jumping, skipping, or beating very fast	Sad or crying for "no reason"
Changes in desire for sex or way sex feels	Unusual or intense dreams

Angry or irritable

Any other concern not on this list

On a scale of 1 (awful) to 10 (wonderful), how are you doing right now? If things are not so good, what would help?

Please tell us about anything else that is worrying you or about any information you want.

(From a tool devised by Linda Glenn, CNM, Portland, OR, based on the Healthy Pregnancy Questions)

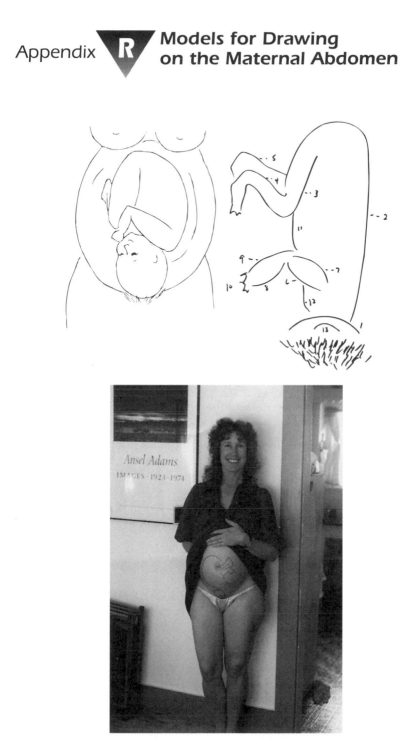

Appendix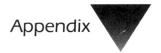

Sample Birth Plan

BIRTH PLAN

1. How have you tried to prepare yourself for labor?
2. What do you think labor will be like?
3. How much pain do you think you will have in labor? Why do you think it will be like that?
4. How long do you think your labor will last? Why do you think it will be that long?
5. What kind of help do you think you will want to deal with the pain of labor?
6. Please list the people you want to be with you in labor. How is each related to you?
7. Are these people welcome to be at the birth also?
8. What do you want your support person to do for you when you are in labor?
9. What is most scary to you about being in labor and giving birth?
10. What is most important to you about this birth?
11. How do you feel about:
    a. Monitoring the baby during labor?
    b. An IV?
    c. The midwife breaking your bag of water?
    d. Using breathing and relaxation techniques to help you through the contractions?
    e. Medication to relieve pain during labor?
    f. An epidural anesthetic to take away the pain of labor?
12. If you had a baby before, did anything happen that might affect you during labor this time?
13. What else about you and how you are likely to act in labor would be helpful for us to know?
14. Is there anything about the people who will be with you in labor that we should know?

Suggestions for What to Bring to the Hospital with You

1. Bring 1 or 2 pillows from home. We have lots but they don't bend in the right places.
2. Bring a few t-shirts, nighties, or large blouses to labor in. They feel better than hospital gowns.
3. Think about bringing . . .
    a. A tape recorder to record your baby's first cry.
    b. A birthday cake. Bake it ahead of time and put it in the freezer until you go into labor.

Appendix ▼T Preparing Children for Childbirth

HOW DOES THE BABY GET OUT? (AND HOW DID HE GET IN THERE ANYWAY?)

Young children who are expecting a new baby in their family are probably more open than they will ever be again to listening to their parents tell them about the "birds and the bees." Although it will probably be easier now than when they are teen-agers, a few tips may help you avoid some tough situations even now:

Relax!

Probably the most important thing you can do is to show your child *by your attitude* that you consider sexuality a natural beautiful part of life. Remember, questions your child asks about this subject are no different to her than any of her other questions. How does the moon keep from falling is no different to her than how babies start; she doesn't yet understand the adult taboos surrounding the subject. So, the best thing you can do is to treat this question with the same calm attitude as any other.

Listen to the Question

A frequent mistake is to answer too much. If your child asks you how the baby will get out, that's what he wants to know—a description of a special tunnel between mommy's legs that can get wider when it's time for the baby's birth—is what he needs; not a detailed description of sperm and eggs. It's usually best to answer only the specific question and then provide a calm, relaxed atmosphere to see if there are any other questions.

For some children, you may need to prompt the questions that they are unable to bring out by themselves. When this is the case, casual conversation about the coming baby will usually provide sufficient opportunity if used carefully. Children's books on the subject may be another aid. Typically, young children who are expecting a new baby in their family are most interested in how the baby will get out. Only later will the question arise concerning how the baby gets in. Discussion of eggs and sperm, and cells and genes are usually appropriate sometime after 7 years of age. Questions about their own bodies are usually the most important to them. They need to know that both boys and girls have wonderful body parts. A girl may be jealous of a boy's penis and boys may be jealous that they won't have breasts when they grow up or be able to become pregnant. All children need to be helped to appreciate the specialness of both their own body and the bodies of the opposite sex. They also need to know that they have always and will always be the same sex. Some little girls fear that they lack a penis because they lost it as a punishment for naughtiness. Some boys fear they will lose it if they are naughty in the future. If your family is uncomfortable with open nudity, pictures may help satisfy your child's need for information about the opposite sex.

If questions center around the birth itself, be alert to their fears related to hospitals and doctors offices—fears of pain and sickness. Be sure these don't become associated with the new baby. Watching animals give birth or using pictures of birth from books may help give them the concrete information they need to conquer their fear of the unknown.

Clear Up Incorrect Information

One of the biggest helps you can give to your child is to clear up any childhood misinformation about sexuality. The best way to do this is to find out what he or she thinks. Answering questions with "How do *you* think it happens?" may be the most enlightening part of your discussion. This will give you the chance to understand misconceptions before replacing them with correct information. Try to avoid telling your child the ideas are totally wrong. You might say, "Oh, that's what I used to think when I was four years old too, but since then I've learned some new things about it . . ." or "What an interesting idea! Let me tell you my idea about how it works. . . ." If he or she doesn't believe your idea or thinks it's peculiar, you might respond with an empathetic "Yes, I used to think it sounded strange too—I always have trouble understanding things I can't see." It's also wise to be aware of several misconceptions so common to this age group that it is a good idea to clear them up even if your child doesn't spontaneously express them:

THE DIGESTIVE FALLACY: BABY IS GROWING IN MOMMY'S TUMMY
This misconception is one of the most common; even many of the children's books use the term tummy or stomach instead of womb or uterus. For some children this can cause serious confusion between how you get pregnant and how you digest food; many eating abnormalities arise during this time because children are frightened of becoming pregnant by eating various foods. Many also fear for the safety and comfort of their new baby as hamburgers and pizza come dropping on his head.

THE AGRICULTURAL FALLACY: BABIES GROW FROM SEEDS LIKE PLANTS
Because of the common description of sperm as seeds, many children associate the baby's beginning with plant seeds, as they're familiar with them. More than one child has tried to swallow watermelon seeds so they can be pregnant too. Using the word sperm instead of seed may help avoid this. Using the word ova instead of egg may also help—this time in preventing the idea of babies hatching like chickens.

BABIES COME FROM . . . THE STORK, THE STORE, THE GARDEN, THE FACTORY, MOTHER'S NAVEL, URETHRA OR ANUS
Although these may be appealing, even charming ideas, they aren't true and can cause confusion in the young child. They also can cause children various worries about their own body. For instance, some children begin to refuse to have bowel movements for fear they might have a baby. These misconceptions need to be replaced with accurate information.

Give Correct Information

Accurate information with correct, but simple terms is the best prevention of problems. Don't worry if you don't know. Your child will learn a lot about problem solving when you just say, "I don't know, but let's find out together," and then check out a book from the local library. There are several books written to supply parents with information they need, and several others written to be read by parents to children. Remember, the best way to use these books is as openers for discussions. Seldom does all of a particular book appeal to any given child, but the pictures are an invaluable aid to your own explanation of things and help elicit your child's questions and misconceptions. The following are some books that may help:

BOOKS FOR PARENTS

The Flight of the Stork by *Anne C. Bernstein,* Dell Publishing Co., 1980.
    A discussion of typical ways in which children understand birth at various ages.
A Child Is Born: The Drama of Life Before Birth by *Axel Ingeman-Sundberg and Claes Wirsen,* Dell Publishers, 1969.
    The classic text of real pictures of unborn babies of various ages. Narrative supplies the parent with needed information. The pictures are good for children as well as parents.

BOOKS FOR PARENTS AND CHILDREN TOGETHER

How Babies Are Made by *Andrew C. Andry and Steven Schepp,* Time Life Books, 1968.
This is probably one of the best books about how babies are made and born written for preschoolers. It begins with pollen and eggs of flowers, goes on to dogs and ends with humans. Paper-cut pictures show accurate anatomy of all of these species, and the combination of accuracy, completeness and simplicity make it ideal for the young child.

Special Delivery, A Book for Kids About Cesarean and Vaginal Birth by *Gayle Cunningham Baker and Vivian M. Montey,* The Chas Franklin Press, 1981.
This is one of the few books available that addresses the experience of Cesarean birth for children. It begins with the anatomical differences between the sexes, and proceeds through intercourse, pregnancy, labor and delivery, and the new baby. Its language tends to be quite technical, and even though explanations are given for the technical terms, there are so many of them that it is likely to be tedious reading for even an older school age child. It will probably have little appeal to a preschooler, but it may give the parent hints on how to explain a Cesarean birth to their child.

How You Were Born by *Joanna Cole,* William Morrow & Company, 1984.
An excellent book for preschool through early school age. Preschoolers may not yet be interested in some of the discussion about sperm and egg, but if they are, the material is presented very clearly. It has lovely pictures of babies at all stages before and after birth. The language is very clear and specific and care is taken to clear up confusions common to this age group.

Gabriel's Very First Birthday by *Sherrie Farrel,* Pipeline Books, 1976.
This book consists of actual photographs starting with pregnancy and ending with breastfeeding. A home delivery assisted by a midwife is depicted, including excellent photographs of the baby at various stages of birth. It does not include making love, but for many children this age, that is not yet an area of interest.

The True Story of How Babies Are Made by *Per Holm Knudsen,* Childrens Press, 1973.
This book uses cartoon-like, but anatomically correct characters; it begins by showing a man and woman making love, and proceeds to show the inside of the woman which now has a cartoon-like baby growing larger page by page. It then shows the baby being born and breastfeeding. Male and female anatomical characteristics are accurate enough to be helpful, although the newborn lacks a cord and placenta. Some may be offended by the total nudity of the figures, but for others, the cartoon-like characteristics help make it less intimidating than actual photographs. Most children will find the pictures quite amusing.

Mom and Dad and I Are Having a Baby by *Maryann P. Malecki,* Pennypress, 1982.
This is an excellent book for a school aged child who will be present at a home delivery. It is told by a child in detail that is probably more than a preschooler would be interested in. It is also quite specific to a home delivery. The hand-drawn pictures are very realistic and the narrative addresses the issues that will be of importance to older children attending the birth, particularly a home birth. Although the book is generally quite accurate and perceptive in addressing issues from a child's point of view, the word "tummy" is frequently used instead of "womb" or "uterus," and may add to the frequent confusion of young children regarding the relation of the stomach to pregnancy.

How Was I Born? by *Lennart Nilsson,* Delacorte Press.
This is the children's version of *A Child Is Born.* The pictures, particularly the world famous pictures of the baby before birth are wonderful. The text is good in suggesting ways of phrasing certain thoughts to the child, but would be too complicated for most preschool children if read directly.

Where Do Babies Come From? by *Margaret Sheffield,* Knopf, 1975.
This is a very accurate and complete account of how babies are made and born. It is illustrated with close-to-photographic art which is quite esthetically pleasing. The narrative would be appropriate for either preschoolers or school age children. Both the narrative and pictures are accurate and complete, including the specific kinds of details that are important to children.

Making Babies: An Open Family Book for Parents and Children Together by *Sara Bonnett Stein,* Walker and Company, 1974.

An excellent book with good full page photographs of animals and people. Pictures of pregnant women, and babies before and after birth as well as young boys and girls showing their anatomical differences are supplemented by photographs of dogs making love, being born and breastfeeding. Probably the best feature of the book is the combination of simple narrative for children with the opposing page filled with good tips for parents on how to handle the discussion with the child.

Most important, remember, if you're not satisfied with how your discussion goes this time, there will be lots of other opportunities. Just relax, and enjoy the chance to help your child learn about one more of the wonderful things in the life around her!

HELPING YOUR CHILD BECOME A BIG SISTER OR BROTHER

A first child is the center of his or her parents' lives. It's not always easy to move over and share the limelight with an uninvited new baby. Here are some hints to help your child become a proud big brother or sister rather than a jealous displaced older child:

Before the Baby Comes

1. **Try to avoid making other major changes in your child's life too close to the coming of the new baby.** If they must be made, be sure to make them considerably before or after the arrival of the new baby so that they won't be associated with the baby. Toilet training and weaning are probably best done 4–6 months after the new baby comes. If they must be done earlier, expect some backsliding when the new baby arrives. Moving to a new bed or bedroom is best done at least 2 months before the baby is expected. This way it won't feel like the new baby is stealing the big siblings' place.

2. **Help your child prepare to keep in touch with mother while she's in the hospital.** Remember, it's not really the new baby that bothers children; it's what they perceive as the loss of their parents' time and attention (spelled L O V E to the child). This starts while the mother is in the hospital. The child can be helped to prepare for this by:

   a. *Learning to use the telephone and talking to mother that way.*

   b. *A trip to the hospital to actually see where mother will be; a visit to the gift shop or lunch in the hospital cafeteria may add excitement to the outing.*

   c. *Pre-recording tapes of mother reading bedtime stories or singing favorite songs.*

   d. *Preparing little presents or notes from mother, to be opened one-a-day. This will be a nice reminder of mother and help count the days til her return.*

   e. *A letter in the mailbox with a little picture or sticker for children who are intrigued by mail.*

   f. *If you're expecting a Cesarean birth, be sure to include in your preparations some pictures or at least a description of the IV tubing, catheter, and abdominal dressing. Such contraptions can be pretty frightening when they're attached to your mother.*

3. **Help your child take part in the preparations.** Let her pick out some of the baby's clothes. Let him help arrange some of the baby's furniture. Help your child select and wrap a gift to the new baby especially from the big brother or sister. Be sure to include some preparations to help the child understand that mother will be leaving for a few days. Letting her help pack the suitcase (including, of course, a picture of the older child) will help to make it more real. A chance to come to mother's prenatal exam and maybe hear the baby's heartbeat can be very exciting. Doing prenatal exercises with mom can be fun too. Be sure your child knows the person who will be caring for him, and try to arrange with this person to continue as many of your child's familiar routines as possible while you're gone. Leave a picture of mom in his bedroom and ask him to take care of something he knows is very important to you while you're gone (watering the plants usually works well).

229

4. **Help prepare your child for what a new baby will really be like.** Pretend play of what it will be like after the baby comes is very effective. Using a favorite doll (or buying one especially for the occasion), play act how it will be when the baby cries, or is hungry or tired. Practicing with diapers or bottles with the doll will give the child a real feel for what is to come. Deciding together what the older child will do when mom or dad needs to take care of the baby will help give the child a sense of power. Maybe the child will feed or change her own "baby" doll, or maybe reading a favorite book while cuddling next to mother and the baby will be the best thing. Books written especially for new brothers and sisters also provide an excellent way to prepare children for a new baby. This is usually a perfect time to relook at your child's baby pictures with her and to reminisce about how she looked and acted as a new baby. Remember to include how careful you had to be with her and to stress that there were lots of things she couldn't do at first. This conversation can lead quite naturally into a discussion about what the new baby will look like (including the umbilicus and lack of teeth) and what he'll be able to do (cry, sleep, see, hear, feel). Maybe most important is what he won't be able to do (like play games with his big sister), and how, over time, he'll learn to do these wonderful things because he is lucky enough to have a big sister who can teach him. The best preparation, of course, is to "borrow" a new baby to babysit for a few hours.
5. **Keep the emphasis not on the new baby, but on the fact that the child will be becoming a big brother or sister and growing older.** You might plan a Big Brother or Sister Celebration when the new baby comes home to celebrate their new status. This might be the time to initiate new privileges of growing older (maybe being able to stay up 15 minutes longer or some other "grown-up privilege").

While Mother Is in the Hospital

Remember, while mother is in the hospital, your child is more likely to be experiencing the absence of mother than the presence of a new baby. For many children, this is the first time they have been away from their mothers, and their reaction is usually a direct reaction to this separation. Signs of anger, fear or regression are common, particularly if the stay in the hospital is very long. Sometimes these reactions, originally toward the separation, become transferred to the new baby. Here are some things you can do to help:

1. **Make efforts to keep contact between mother and child.** This is where your previous planning will pay dividends. Now is the time to use the pre-recorded tapes of mother's voice, the gifts left by her, the cards in the mailbox. Most important is as much visiting to the hospital as possible and use of the telephone.
2. **Make efforts to start a positive introduction between your child and the new baby.** This is the time to send home a present (bought beforehand) from the baby to his big brother or sister. A congratulations card from the baby through the mail (or at least planted in the mailbox to make it quicker) may also be an excellent introduction. Different hospitals have different policies about children seeing and/or holding their new baby siblings. If at all possible, see if your older child can see and touch his new sibling while visiting mother at the hospital. Letting your older child make some of the phone calls to announce the new arrival can make him feel an important part of things. Having her name with yours on the birth announcement can be fun too.

After the Baby Comes

Finally, the new baby comes home! A joy to all? Well, maybe. . . .

1. **Be prepared for a less-than-friendly reception.** No matter how well you have prepared your child, the initial encounter may be difficult—or the initial encounter may be fine, only to be followed a few weeks or months later by the calm announcement "Let's give him back to the hospital now!" If you are not taken by surprise by these reactions, you will be in a better position to help your child adjust to his or her new sibling. Sometimes a young child reacts directly toward the baby by hitting or grabbing away his bottle; more often it is indirect, often by over-rough

"loves," or more demanding behavior or whining. Many children who were potty trained or weaned before the new baby, seem to forget these skills once the newcomer arrives. After all, if you saw all those adults saying how cute the new baby was when he cried and wet his pants and sucked a bottle, wouldn't you try it too? The best response to these behaviors is no response at all, only increased attention to your child at other times. Often it helps to say out loud what he is saying in his mind "Oh, would you like to pretend you're a little baby too? OK, here, I'll give you your bottle; then later you'll decide to be my big boy again."

2. **Help him or her see the advantages of being a "big" boy or girl.** Comments such as: "Oh, you want to be a little baby now; let me rock you; then when you decide to be a big boy again, you can help me make cookies—babies are too little to do that!"

3. **Provide help for the tough times.** Your older child is most likely to experience difficulties when you first come home, and later at times when the baby needs the most attention. Try to have someone other than mother carry the new baby home. Be sure to make the first fuss over the big sibling and how mother has missed him. There will be time later to all talk about and look at the new baby. Planning ahead may help alleviate some of the later problems, especially at feeding times. Some children enjoy feeding their baby while you feed yours—and changing their baby while you change yours. Providing a baby doll, bottle, and a few disposable diapers (handkerchiefs work well) ahead of time may be a big help. A special "feeding time" box, placed next to the spot where baby is fed and filled with special toys that can be used only during feeding time can be great fun. A new little surprise toy might be placed there every once in a while to be discovered during feeding time. Keeping a stool next to the changing table so she can get high enough to see and help may help her feel more a part of the family. Helping him to hold, hug and talk to the baby will help too. A special "big brother chair" where he can sit and have the baby safely laid in his arms will help set safe limits for holding the new baby without making the older child feel left out. Even running errands may help a small child feel important.

4. **Help the visitors pay special attention to the big brother or sister.** A word beforehand to grandparents and others will help them remember to greet the big brother or sister first and let *them* be the ones to take the visitors into the baby's room. Keeping a hidden cache of inexpensive "Big Brother or Sister Presents," which can be discreetly handed to the visitor to give with the baby gift often help considerably. Show the visitors not only pictures of the new baby but also some of the big sibling when he or she was a baby.

5. **Help the big brother or sister recognize and accept both their positive and negative feelings toward the baby.** Children usually begin to understand the concept of jealousy about the age of 4 or 5. Younger children will understand the concept of anger. Saying out loud what the child is feeling inside can be very helpful, "I know it makes you feel mad that I'm feeding baby instead of drawing with you. Baby is so little that she doesn't know how to wait yet like big boys do. Thank you for waiting. As soon as I'm done feeding her, I'll draw some pictures with you."

   It's also important to tell the child what kinds of things she can and cannot do when she feels mad, "I see that you are feeling angry with baby right now. That's OK, and if you want to show me how angry you are, you can punch that pillow as hard as you want, but you can't hit baby." Protect your older sibling (and your new baby) by playing it safe. Lower the crib mattress so the big sibling can't try to pick the baby up, and never leave a child under 10 alone with the baby—even for just a minute!

6. **Schedule "private time" with your older child.** Just knowing that mom or dad will be all theirs at 6:00 to do "big boy things" that babies are too little for can help tremendously.

7. **Help big brothers and sisters recognize the growth and development of the new baby.** Children are often disappointed to discover that the new baby isn't really much of a playmate. Preparation for what a baby is really like will help some, but even well prepared children won't understand what it will *really* be like to have a baby in the house until the actual arrival. Once the baby is home, it helps to have the older sibling watching for each new development. Let *him* be the first to break the news that the baby smiled for the first time—at his big brother, of course! Show her

how to let the baby grab her finger; teach him to hold a bright shiny object about a foot away from the baby's eyes and coach the baby to begin to slowly follow the object. Big siblings will love to make a baby book for themselves, "Baby and Me," complete with dates of when the baby first smiled at the older sibling, pictures of the two together and anecdotes about different things the older sibling discovered about the baby (the first smile, the first reach, the first laugh). It will help them appreciate and be a part of the baby's small developmental gains even before he can be a good ball partner.

These are all little tips that you can use to help your child become a Big Sister or Big Brother, but the most important thing is just to make sure that your child understands that you still love him just as much as ever, and your love is enough for two!

Appendix U

Words Found to be Difficult by Women With Low Literacy Skills

Pamphlet	Number of Women		
	Three	Four	Five
Nutrition	represents physical	amniotic pregnant placenta sensible	
Smoking	anxiety benefits breathing bronchitis cigarettes concerns discomfort experiencing inhaled increases nerves nervousness normal oxygen pressure supply unpleasant	associated carbon monoxide especially nicotine prone quitting symptoms	accumulate pneumonia significantly thus
Fitness	aerobic activities awareness complex discovered efficiency especially essential flatten hollowed immediate machine perform physically prescription remarkable response satisfying uterus utmost	abdomen capacities component jar ligament neutral organs pelvis revitalizing stimulus vitality	buttocks groin essence individualistic sensitive stitch

(Reprinted with permission from Farkas, C.S., Glenday, P.G., O'Connor, P.J., & Schmeltzer, J. (1987). Evaluation of the readability of prenatal health education materials. *Canadian Journal of Public Health, 78*, 377.)

Appendix V Checklist for Printed Material

TITLE OF MATERIAL:

Organization

1. The cover is attractive. It indicates the core content and intended audience.
2. Desired behavior changes are stressed. "Need to know" information is stressed.
3. Not more than three or four main points are presented.
4. Headers and summaries are used to show organization and provide message repetition.
5. A summary that stresses what to do is included.

Writing Style

6. The writing is in conversational style, active voice.
7. There is little or no technical jargon.
8. Text is vivid and interesting. Tone is friendly.

Appearance

9. Pages or sections appear uncluttered. Ample white spaces.
10. Lowercase letters used (capitals used only where grammatically needed).
11. There is a high degree of contrast between the print and the paper.
12. Print size is at least 12 point, serif type, and no stylized letters.
13. Illustrations are simple—preferably line drawings.
14. Illustrations serve to amplify the text.

Appeal

15. The material is culturally, gender, and age appropriate.
16. The material closely matches the logic, language, and experience of the intended audience.
17. Interaction is invited via questions, responses, suggested action, etc.

(Reprinted with permission from Doak, C.C., Doak, L.G., & Root, J.H. (1996). *Teaching patients with low literacy skills.* Philadelphia: J.B. Lippincott, 43.)

Appendix W

Sample Patient Education Material*

QUESTIONS THAT PREGNANT WOMEN OFTEN ASK

How often should my baby move?

Babies should move at least 10 times every 12 hours. Most babies move much more often than that. Some even move hundreds of times each day.

If you think your baby might not be moving enough:
- Drink 2 glasses of something right away—like water, milk, or juice.
- Eat if you have not eaten in the last 2 hours.

Then lie down and count how many times the baby moves in 1 hour. If the baby moves 5 times in an hour, or if the baby moves 5 times before the hour is over, you can stop.

If the baby doesn't move 5 times in an hour . . .

Call 000-0000 and ask to speak to the nurse–midwife. She may ask you to come to the hospital to have a nonstress test. This test is also called an NST.

Remember that the baby should not stop moving when labor begins.

Is it OK to have sex when I am pregnant?

Almost any kind of sexual activity is all right in pregnancy if there are no problems and the mother-to-be wants to have it. Only blowing into the vagina of a pregnant woman is dangerous.

It is OK to make love or have sex as long as:
- The mother-to-be wants to do it.
- It doesn't cause her any pain or discomfort.
- She has no vaginal bleeding.
- Her water hasn't broken.
- Labor hasn't started.

Sometimes couples are afraid that sex might hurt the unborn baby. They might also think that having sex is too noisy for the baby. If the baby moves while they are making love, some people think the baby doesn't like what is happening.

We can't say for sure what the baby is thinking or feeling inside the uterus. But we do know that it is pretty noisy inside the womb already. The mother's heart beats, food moves through her intestines, and air goes into her lungs. Think what it sounds like when she drinks a glass of water!

As far as we know, if there are no problems and the mother-to-be is interested, making love during pregnancy is a nice way for couples to show their love for each other.

What should I know about preeclampsia (toxemia)?

Preeclampsia is a word that means a pregnant woman has high blood pressure. Her urine may also have protein in it, and her face may be swollen. Preeclampsia is dangerous because it can lead to convulsions (seizures). The mother-to-be could have a stroke.

Your blood pressure is checked at each clinic visit to look for preeclampsia. Your urine is tested for protein. Your weight is checked because weight gain may be the first sign of swelling.

---

* Credit to Linda Wheeler, CNM.

Other signs of preeclampsia to look for are:
- Headaches that won't go away, even when you lie down or take Tylenol
- Spots in front of your eyes that won't go away
- Pain in your breast bone or chest
- Pain below your ribs on the right side

If you have any of these signs, be sure to call the nurse–midwife at 000-0000.

Should I be scared if I feel contractions before my due date?

Contractions that you feel before the baby is due can be a sign of premature labor. Babies born too early can be very sick.

If you have more than 6 contractions in an hour *and* you have more than 3 weeks to wait until your baby is due, *then* drink 2 glasses of something (water, milk and juice are good choices) *and* eat if you haven't eaten in 2 hours.

If you still have 6 contractions in an hour or the contractions come more often, *call the nurse–midwife.*

Other signs of premature labor include:
- Backache that won't go away
- Pressure that you feel low in your abdomen
- Cramping
- Change in discharge from your vagina

Call the nurse–midwife if you notice these things.

Appendix X — Postpartum Patient History Form for Patients to Complete

1. Please check if you are having problems with any of the following:
   Bleeding
   Pain
   Vaginal discharge
   Feeling tired
   Controlling urine, gas, or bowel movement
   Burning when urinating (peeing)
   Pain when having sex
2. Please check how often you find yourself (not often, pretty often, very often):
   Irritable
   Crying
   Not able to sleep
   Overwhelmed
   Happy
   Sad
   Depressed
   Exhausted
   Scared
   Excited
   Tired
   Not eating well
   Content
   Hard to get along with
   Angry
   Worried
   Anxious
3. On a scale of 1 to 10, with 1 being awful and 10 being wonderful, how do you think things are going with your partner?
4. On a scale of 1 to 10, how do you think things are going with you and the baby?
5. On a scale of 1 to 10, how do you think things are going with your partner and the baby?
6. Please rate how easy you think it is to take care of your baby. Let 1 be very difficult and 10 be very easy.
7. What is most helpful to you now?
8. What would you like to have more help with?
9. What is hardest for you now?
10. Please check the things that are most stressful for you right now.
    Difficult baby
    Relationship with partner
    Relationship with family
    Money
    Housing
    Child care
    Breastfeeding
    Returning to work
    Getting pregnant
    My weight
    Having sex
    Other things

11. When you left the hospital, how were you feeding the baby?
    Breastfeeding
    Bottlefeeding
    How are you feeding the baby now?
    Breast
    Bottle
12. If you have had sex since the baby was born, please answer the following questions.
    Have you had a new sex partner since the baby was born?
    Did you have any pain?
    Were you ready to have sex?
    Did you have any problems with feeling dry?
    Did you notice any difference having sex now compared to having sex before you got pregnant?
    Has your partner said anything about sex being different?
13. What are you using/planning to use for birth control? Why is this a good method for you?
14. What medicine have you taken since the baby was born?
15. Have you made any visits to an emergency room or clinic for something other than a regular check-up since the baby was born?
16. Are you smoking?
17. Have you drunk any alcohol since the baby was born?
18. Please list any drugs you have had since the baby was born (include marijuana).
19. Are you working or planning to work?
20. Please check if you would like information about any of the following.
    Parenting an infant
    Parenting children of other ages
    Weight-loss ideas
    Drug and alcohol programs
    Stop-smoking programs
    Anger-control programs
    Support groups for women who have been abused
    Counseling
    Something else
21. What questions would you like to get answered today?

Appendix Y Suggestions for Discussing Condom Use with a Man

Talk about using condoms ahead of time. This may be both difficult and awkward, but it is better than bringing up the subject in the heat of lovemaking. The best case scenario would be a grateful partner who is delighted that someone else brought the subject up. The next best scenario is a partner who is not quite delighted but who is ready to listen. You can emphasize:

a. You are showing respect for him by not wanting to take any chances.

b. He has a chance to show respect for you.

c. This is new sex, not second class sex. Condoms don't have to be unpleasant—they can be fun, erotic, playful.

d. Think of the condom as part of lovemaking rather than interruption or bother.

The worst case scenario is a partner who thinks safer sex is unnecessary, and says "I'm not gonna use no condom," "I don't need a condom," or "You gotta be crazy." Imagine that you are in this situation. What could you say in response?

You might buy different kinds of condoms ahead of time, or visit clinics that hand them out free. Invite a friend to go with you if you are embarrassed. Invite your partner to go with you. Set aside some time to play with them to find out which kind would work best. Be aware that condoms available without cost often do not contain nonoxynol-9. Here is some information that might be helpful.

a. Size: While condoms are very elastic (try blowing one up) and adjust to a variety of penis sizes, there are a few brands for men with smaller or larger penises. If one brand does not fit, try another.

b. Lubrication: Some condoms are lubricated and some are not. Lubricated condoms are thought to be less likely to break. Unfortunately, lubricated condoms often have a strong rubber taste and are, therefore, not suitable for oral sex. Lubricated condoms may be coated with a chemical known as nonoxynol-9. It provides extra protection against the AIDS virus, but some people are allergic to it. Use a condom coated with nonoxynol-9 if you can. This ingredient is listed on the outside of the condom package when present.

Use a water-soluble lubricant such as Astro Glide if you need more lubrication on the condom. If you use other lubricants such as Vaseline, baby oil, Nivea Cream, hand lotion, massage oil, or Crisco, the condom is more likely to break.

c. The condom's tip: Condoms come with or without a tip to hold the semen (cum). Some people who like oral sex don't like the tip. Others don't mind it. Condoms with a tip on the end are less likely to break than those without a tip. If you use a condom without a tip, leave a ¼-inch space at the end of the condom as it goes on to the penis. This leaves space for the cum when the man ejaculates. When you put a condom on, squeeze the tip or the ¼-inch at the end so that no air is left in the condom. Friction can make the bubble pop.

d. Thickness: The thicker the condom, the less likely it is to break. But the thicker it is, the less feeling there is. Experiment to find which one is right for you. Thin is usually good for oral sex, but remember that anal sex increases the chances that a condom will break. Thicker is better—at least it is safer.

e. Special features: Condoms come in different colors and some even glow in the dark. Some are ribbed to provide extra feeling, and some are flavored with mint or fruit, including Wild Strawberry, to taste good. Flavored condoms may also contain nonoxynol-9.

f. Storage: Condoms often come with an expiration date. Don't confuse it with the date of manufacture. High temperatures can cause the condom to break. Avoid putting condoms in the glove compartment of your car on a hot day or in direct sunlight. You may have heard you shouldn't keep them in your wallet. But a recent study showed no increase in breakage after carrying the condom in a wallet for a long time. Although they may not be ideal, wallets, shoes and the inside of a bra can be okay places for a condom.

g. Other helpful information:

Use latex condoms rather than sheepskin condoms. Latex condoms are cheaper, protect against the AIDS virus, and are less likely to break.

If you know you are going to have sex, loosen the wrapping on the condom as you go to bed (if you have sex in bed) to avoid fumbling at an inopportune time.

Use each condom one time only.

Open the condom carefully. Tearing or long fingernails can damage it.

Don't test it by stretching or inflating it.

Leave a paper towel and wastebasket by your bed. Put the used condom on the paper towel when you are finished with it. Later, put it in the waste basket. Do not flush the condom down the toilet.

Leave a damp cloth and a towel by the bed. The cloth can wipe off any lubricant if oral sex is desired and you are not using a flavored condom. Later, the damp cloth can be used to freshen each other up.

Talking about condoms can lead to a better communication about sex in general.

If you are new to using condoms, some suggest waiting until you are close to coming before you put the condom on. If you do this, be sure to keep the penis away from the vagina since the pre-cum may contain HIV and sperm. Squeeze the air out of the tip of the condom if it is the kind with the tip. If the condom does not have a tip, squeeze about ¼ inch of the blunt end so that there will be space for the cum.

Uncircumcised men (or their partner) should pull back the foreskin before putting the condom on.

Check the condom periodically to make sure it is on.

If you are going to have oral sex and the condom is not flavored, wipe it off with a damp wash cloth after putting it on. Experiment with different brands to find the one that is least objectionable or get a kind with a flavor you find pleasant.

If you are going to have anal sex, use lots of water-based lubricant and don't let the condom dry out. It might break.

After coming, pull the penis and condom out before your partner has lost his erection. Have your partner hold on to the base of the penis as it comes out so that the condom does not come off and semen does not spill out.

Appendix Z ▼ Relief Measures for the Common Discomforts of Pregnancy

1. **Backache**

    Distinguish between musculoskeletal strain, sciatica, and a sacroiliac joint (SI) problem (often sharp and involving one side of the ilium).

    For musculoskeletal strain

    Pillow in lumbar area while sitting, massage, ice or heat, chiropractic, footstool under one foot while standing, pillow between knees when lying on side

    For SI dysfunction

    Nonelastic sacroiliac belt placed after performing one of the exercises below (improvement will be slow), wedge-shaped pillow under abdomen when side-lying, trochanteric belt worn below the belly at the femoral heads to increase joint stability.

    Exercise 1: Lie supine, pull bended knee toward body with hands while pushing with knee; alternate knees and repeat up to 15 to 20 times daily

    Exercise 2: Bend the knee and hip on one side and put the knee into the ipsilateral axilla. Alternate several times.

2. **Breast tenderness**

    Good bra, don't touch, careful lovemaking

3. **Carpal tunnel syndrome** (Tingling, numbness, stiffness, burning, swelling, weakness, pain, decreased dexterity, nocturnal awakening)

    Rest the affected hand, ice, elevate, wrist splints, rolled washcloth placed in the palmar surface of the hand, avoid repetitive wrist activities, mild analgesia

4. **Constipation**

    Increase fluids, increase dietary fiber, drink prune juice, exercise regularly, drink a glass of warm water in AM

5. **Dependent edema**

    Bed rest for 24 hours

6. **Faintness**

    Change positions slowly, avoid dehydration, avoid lying flat on back, avoid prolonged standing or sitting

7. **Fatigue**

    Reassure that it usually passes by 16 weeks and, no matter how much rest and sleep she gets, the fatigue remains; therefore, rearrange responsibilities, become a couch potato, and throw away the guilt

    Decrease activities, adjust fluid intake at night to decrease the number of times it is necessary to get up to urinate

8. **Flatulence**

    Peppermint candy, parsley

9. **Headaches**

    Head/shoulder/face massage, acupressure, hot or cold compresses, rest, biofeedback, progressive relaxation, warm bath, meditation, aromatherapy, analgesia

10. **Heartburn**

    Small, frequent meals; papaya (fresh, dried, canned juice, enzymes), slippery elm bark throat lozenges, raw almonds after meals, don't bend over, sleep with head elevated, half a lemon in cool water, antacids

11. **Hemorrhoids**

    Freeze cotton balls/4×4s soaked in witch hazel, apply Tucks, take sitz baths, avoid constipation

    Peel a potato and cut a piece about ¼ inch in diameter and insert into rectum allowing it to be expelled with next bowel movement

12. **Insomnia**
    Warm bath, hot drink, good book, TV, avoid daytime nap
13. **Leg cramps**
    Decrease phosphate in diet by drinking no more than 2 glasses of milk per day, massage affected muscle, don't point toes, try calf stretch exercises, keep legs warm, exercise/walk, magnesium tabs: 122 mg every AM and 244 mg every PM While studies have not proven calcium tablets to be effective, they are widely used (1.5 to 2.0 g daily), and ancedotal reports support their use.
14. **Leukorrhea**
    Evaluate for vaginitis and STDs
    Good perineal hygiene, change panties as often as needed to stay dry
15. **Nausea/vomiting**
    Acupressure including wrist bands, 10 gtts peppermint spirits in half a glass of water, raspberry leaf tea, potato chips and lemonade, continuous nibbling, hard candy, eat what you want when you want it, a snack at bedtime, keep food at bedside and eat each time there is a nocturnal trip to the bathroom, drink liquids between meals rather than with meals, lie down, sip on a carbonated beverage or carbonated water, pyridoxine (vitamin B_6) 10 to 25 mg tid, meclizine (Antivert) 25 mgm tid
    Try drinking ½ cup of the Morning Sickness Milkshake every 30 minutes (Courtesy of Kate Davidson, CNM, Salem, OR)
        1 quart of milk or yogurt
        frozen fruit
        4 eggs (advise of potential danger of salmonella)
        sweetener and/or cinnamon or nutmeg
16. **Round ligament pain**
    Consider appendicitis, ovarian cyst, placental separation, inguinal hernia
    Bend over, warm compresses, avoid sudden movement, avoid twisting, raise knee to chest on affected side
17. **Sciatica**
    Massage, chiropractic
18. **Skin rashes**
    Ice, diphenhydramine (Benadryl) 25 mg po for itching, dermatology referral
19. **Symphysis pubis pain**
    Maternity girdle/sacroiliac belt
20. **Urinary frequency**
    Avoid caffeine
21. **Varicosities**
    TEDS/support stockings applied before sitting up/getting out of bed, calensonia root capsules, perineal pad inside panties if vulvar varicosities

REMEMBER

1. There are little data to support most of the recommendations to relieve the common discomforts of pregnancy.
2. What works for one woman may not work for another.
3. Uncertain dosage and product contamination are possible with herbs.

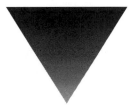

Index

Note: Page numbers followed by "b" indicate boxed material; page numbers followed by "f" indicate figures; page numbers followed by "t" indicate tabular material.

A

Ectopic pregnancy, 35
    classic symptoms in, 104
    fear of death in, 104
    IUD use and, 34
    pelvic inflammatory disease and, 37
    RhIg following, 72
    suspicion of, 104
Edema
    in preeclampsia, 101
    in pregnancy, 109
Education history, initial prenatal, 54
Emergency, procedure for, 88
Emotional abuse. *See* Physical/emotional abuse
Encephalocele, maternal serum alfa fetoprotein levels in, 135
Engorgement
    differential diagnosis of, 153
    treatment of, 153
Environmental exposure history, 14
    from hobbies, 55
    initial prenatal, 50
    initial prenatal visit, 50
    occupational prenatal, 53
    preconception, 26
    preconception history, 14
Enzyme immunoassay (EIA), for HIV infection, 81
Epidural anesthesia, 143
Epilepsy, preconception history, 7
Erythema infectiosum. *See* Parvovirus B19 (erythema infectiosum; Fifth's Disease)
Erythromycin
    for chlamydia trachomatis, 69, 70b
    for mastitis, 152b
Estimated date of delivery (EDD), 32–33
    gestation calculators in, 33
    menstrual frequency and duration in, 33
    Naegele's rule in, 32–33
Ethnic background
    client terms for, 47
    cultural sensitivity to, 46–47, 48b
    initial prenatal history, 45–49
    preconception history, 4
    special blood tests and, 84
Exercise
    preconception, 25
    prenatal assessment and recommendations, 56
Exophthalmus, prenatal, 61
Expectant mother, honoring, 144–145
Extremities, initial prenatal examination of, 66

F
Family constellation, in prenatal history, 52–53
Family history
    of cancer, 4, 166, 167
    of father, 4